COLLABORATIVE AND INDIGENOUS MENTAL HEALTH THERAPY

This book examines a collaboration between traditional Māori healing and clinical psychiatry. Comprised of transcribed interviews and detailed meditations on practice, it demonstrates how bicultural partnership frameworks can augment mental health treatment by balancing local imperatives with sound and careful psychiatric care. In the first chapter, Māori healer Wiremu NiaNia outlines the key concepts that underpin his worldview and work. He then discusses the social, historical, and cultural context of his relationship with Allister Bush, a child and adolescent psychiatrist. The main body of the book comprises chapters that each recount the story of one young person and their family's experience of Māori healing from three or more points of view: those of the psychiatrist, the Māori healer, and the young person and other family members who participated in and experienced the healing. With a foreword by Sir Mason Durie, this book is essential reading for psychologists, social workers, nurses, therapists, psychiatrists, and students interested in bicultural studies.

Wiremu NiaNia was apprenticed as a child to a spiritual healer of the NiaNia whānau. In 2005 he became the cultural therapist at Te Whare Mārie, the Māori mental health service at Capital Coast District Health Board. He is now an independent healer, writer, and consultant.

Allister Bush is a child and adolescent psychiatrist at Te Whare Mārie, the Māori mental health service in Porirua, and at Health Pasifika (integrated Pacific mental health service, Capital Coast District Health Board).

David Epston is an honorary clinical lecturer at University of Melbourne and an affiliate faculty member at North Dakota State University.

Writing Lives
Ethnographic Narratives

Series Editors Arthur P. Bochner, Carolyn Ellis
(University of South Florida) and Tony E. Adams
(Northeastern Illinois University)

Writing Lives: Ethnographic Narratives publishes narrative representations of qualitative research projects. The series editors seek manuscripts that blur the boundaries between humanities and social sciences. We encourage novel and evocative forms of expressing concrete lived experience, including autoethnographic, literary, poetic, artistic, visual, performative, critical, multivoiced, conversational, and co-constructed representations. We are interested in ethnographic narratives that depict local stories; employ literary modes of scene setting, dialogue, character development, and unfolding action; and include the author's critical reflections on the research and writing process, such as research ethics, alternative modes of inquiry and representation, reflexivity, and evocative storytelling. Proposals and manuscripts should be directed to abochner@usf.edu, cellis@usf.edu, or aeadams3@neiu.edu.

Other volumes in this series include:

Bullied
Tales of Torment, Identity, and Youth
Keith Berry

Evocative Autoethnography
Writing Lives and Telling Stories
Arthur P. Bochner and Carolyn Ellis

Staring at the Park
A Poetic Autoethnographic Inquiry
Jane Speedy

Transcribing Silence
Culture, Relationships, and Communication
Kristine L. Muñoz

For a full list of titles in this series, please visit **www.routledge.com/Writing-Lives-Ethnographic-Narratives/book-series/WLEN**

COLLABORATIVE AND INDIGENOUS MENTAL HEALTH THERAPY

Tātaihono — Stories of Māori Healing and Psychiatry

Wiremu NiaNia, Allister Bush, and David Epston

Routledge
Taylor & Francis Group
NEW YORK AND LONDON

First published 2017
by Routledge
605 Third Avenue, New York, NY 10017

and by Routledge
2 Park Square, Milton Park, Abingdon, Oxon, OX14 4RN

Routledge is an imprint of the Taylor & Francis Group, an informa business

Library of Congress Cataloging in Publication Data
Names: NiaNia, Wiremu, author. | Bush, Allister, author. | Epston, David, author.
Title: Collaborative and indigenous mental health therapy : tātaihono, stories of Māori healing and psychiatry / by Wiremu NiaNia, Allister Bush, and David Epston.
Description: New York : Routledge, 2017. | Includes bibliographical references and index.
Identifiers: LCCN 2016026432 (print) | LCCN 2016046190 (ebook) | ISBN 9781138230286 (hardback) | ISBN 9781138230309 (pbk.) | ISBN 9781315386423 (ebk.) | ISBN 9781315386423 (eBook)
Subjects: LCSH: Māori (New Zealand people)—Mental health services. | Traditional medicine.
Classification: LCC RA790.7.N7 N53 2017 (print) | LCC RA790.7.N7 (ebook) | DDC 362.196/89008999442—dc23
LC record available at https://lccn.loc.gov/2016026432

ISBN: 978-1-138-23028-6 (hbk)
ISBN: 978-1-138-23030-9 (pbk)
ISBN: 978-1-315-38642-3 (ebk)

Typeset in Bembo
by Apex CoVantage, LLC

For Product Safety Concerns and Information please contact our EU representative: GPSR@taylorandfrancis.com
Taylor & Francis Verlag GmbH, Kaufingerstraße 24, 80331 München, Germany.

This book is dedicated to Te Kaihanga and Te Ao Wairua

The names of all young people and their family members referred to in this book have been changed and some other details have been altered to protect their identities. Each of their stories has been shared with their permission.

Winner of the 2014 Ashton Wylie Unpublished Manuscript Award

CONTENTS

FOREWORD

In *Tātaihono* three mental health practitioners—Wiremu, Allister, and David—share their experiences and insights gained by moving outside conventional psychiatric frameworks. Throughout the book first-hand accounts are used to illustrate how unlikely relationships evolved into working partnerships and how those partnerships provided a basis for a comprehensive approach to advancing the health of patients and their families. As a result the trio has been able to articulate a model of care that will be increasingly relevant in a world where global migration and cultural diversity already demand multiple perspectives. The advancement of health, education, economic growth, environmental sustainability, societal equity, and fairness will all require a capacity to share knowledge and learning and to work outside accustomed frameworks.

The model of care that emerges from *Tātaihono* draws on two quite different worldviews—science and indigenous knowledge. Although the two are based on seemingly divergent philosophies, when applied together the divergence can be replaced by a synergy that dwarfs the scope of either acting alone. By straddling mind, body, and spirit *Tātaihono* has been able to reveal the comprehension and skills needed if the combination of the two approaches can augment recovery from stress or illness. Too often mental health treatment and care have focussed exclusively on the mind without due consideration for wairua (spirit), tinana (body), or whānau (family). Similarly traditional indigenous healing has often been largely associated with spiritual renewal, though not necessarily with health gains in other dimensions.

Indigenous approaches are strongly aligned to time-honoured healing methods and in that context are enhanced by time. In contrast, clinical practices place greater emphasis on a readiness to adapt to fresh knowledge; they are enhanced by new discoveries and constantly changing scientific evidence. In that respect, whereas indigenous healers revere old knowledge, medical practitioners are encouraged to use new knowledge to give effect to fresh evidence.

The interface between medical practice and traditional healing has often been a site for frank disagreements, mutual ridicule, and shared loss of respect each for the other. Disputes at the interface reflect differences in the two bodies of knowledge—science and indigenous knowledge—as well as differences in methods of practice, understandings of health, and outcome goals.

Tātaihono also highlights the significance of therapist backgrounds. Engagement in any therapeutic encounter is a two-way process that is shaped by the cultural starting points that each party brings. Rightly, *Tātaihono* is a reminder that therapists need to be conscious of their own cultural perspectives and how those viewpoints might affect treatment and care.

More importantly, however, *Tātaihono* illustrates how those seemingly immovable barriers can be overcome without either approach forfeiting basic tenets. Three principles for collaboration stand out. First, the temptation to understand the other by using, for example, the tools of science to 'explain' indigenous approaches, or using indigenous worldviews to comprehend scientific approaches, leads nowhere. Mutual respect is necessary. Second, collaboration requires a willingness to acknowledge that neither approach has all the answers. Third, in the end the purpose of any healing process is to benefit the patient, using methods that most align with each case. Therein lies the challenge—to determine which approach is likely to be the most appropriate and whether there is an indication for the application of both in parallel.

Tātaihono makes a significant contribution to the literature. It is testimony to the importance of spirit as a key element in the journey towards mental health and of the benefits derived from the application of two bodies of knowledge.

Mauri Ora.

Sir Mason Durie
Emeritus Professor, Massey University
Palmerston North, New Zealand

PEPEHA

Pepeha	*Wiremu's introduction*
Ka huri taku titiro	As I turn to gaze
Ki ngā puketaumutu a Whakapunake	At the summit hilltops of Whakapunake
E rewatu ana ki te rangi	Extending toward heaven
Ka ari ngā taringa	I hear the splashing
Ki te haruru a te taniwha a Hinekōrako	of Hinekōrako
Ki te hononga a ngā wai	At the coming together
Te Ruakituri me Te Hangaroa	of the Ruakituri and the Hangaroa
Ka takarere atu ki Te Wairoa	Cascading down
Hōnengenenge hōpūpū matangirau	to the turbulent waters of Te Wairoa
Ka pikowai ka puta atu ki te moana	and winding its way to the sea
Ko te iti a Tūhoe i roto o Ngāti Hinehika	It is a descendant of Tūhoe who dwells in the midst of Ngāti Hinehika
E tangi atu nei ki te kohinga wairua	Who grieves for and acknowledges the gathering of the spirits
Āpiti hono tātai hono	Let that which has been joined remain intact
Kia tūturu! Whakamaua kia tina!	
Hui ē, tāiki ē!	It is done!

ABBREVIATIONS

AIM	American Indian Movement
CAF	child, adolescent and family
CT	computed tomography scan
DSM	*Diagnostic and Statistical Manual of Mental Disorders*
EEG	electroencephalogram
EIS	Early Intervention Service
Health Pasifika CAFS	Pacific Child, Adolescent and Family Service
Māori CAFS	Māori Child, Adolescent and Family Service
UNDRIP	United Nations Declaration on the Rights of Indigenous Peoples

1

INTRODUCTION

Wiremu

Tēnā koutou katoa. This is my greeting to you, the reader. I welcome you to our book.

This book is a collection of true stories of Māori healing. The stories show the joining of a traditional cultural approach with the clinical approach of psychiatry and the forging of a working relationship between Allister and me that allowed this to take place.

In this chapter I will explain what the word matekite (seeing sickness or death) means and why I asked Allister if we could write this book together. I go on to talk about three Māori concepts that are intrinsic to all my work: mana (spiritual authority), mauri (life force), and tapu (something sacred or forbidden). In Chapter 2 we will look at the context to this mahi (work). In the stories that follow you will see these concepts in action and how they make a difference to the lives of the young people concerned.

Next, I speak about my background and how I eventually came to be working as a cultural therapist at Te Whare Mārie, the Māori mental health service where Allister and I met. Allister, who is a Pākehā (New Zealander of European descent) psychiatrist, will then tell how he came to be working in a Māori service and will give his account of how we began our work together.

You may wish to bypass all this kōrero (explanation), in which case I would encourage you to go straight to the stories that start in Chapter 3.

Matekite and Healing

I define matekite[1] as a kind of seeing that pertains to sickness and death. But it is a seeing that goes beyond normal human vision. I am descended from a long line of seers, and for me the most influential was my kuia (female elder), Te Awhimate Trainor NiaNia. I will tell you more about her in a moment.

Here is how I explain matekite:

> Mā te kite ka mōhio, mā te mōhio ka kitea he oranga. ('By the seeing, one will have knowledge; by that knowledge, one will find an answer.')

And, of course, you can see that the first three words of this proverb combine to form the word 'matekite'. This saying tells us that this kind of seeing has been part of healing in Māori culture going way back. And the meaning of this proverb relates to the reason I asked Allister if we could write this book together in the first place.

Awareness

We write these stories to show that there is more to Māori culture than just what you see in front of you. Since I was young I have often seen things; heard things; or even felt, tasted, and smelt things that others were unable to see, hear, feel, taste, or smell. If I had been seen by a mental health clinician and they asked me, 'Are you seeing things?' I would have said, 'Yes'.

Consequently, I would be in danger of being misdiagnosed. I could have been labelled as having hallucinations or being psychotic. And I strongly believe this has been a problem for many of our people. When I say this, I'm not suggesting that mental illness doesn't exist. But far too often the wairua side, the spiritual side, has gone unrecognised, which has had very negative outcomes for us as Māori.

In this book, we are inviting you to look outside the box. And if you are a mental health clinician, we are inviting you to look beyond the DSM.[2] We are by no means saying 'abandon it altogether'. But we are declaring there are some matters it cannot explain.

My aim is to produce the kind of awareness that imparts knowledge that can be used to help heal those who are suffering. It is my hope that, armed with this knowledge, we mental health clinicians might make fewer mistakes in terms of diagnosing our people.

Explaining Things

In my mahi there are some matters over which I take particular care. One of these is explaining things to people. I want people to be able to understand what I'm talking about. I want wairuatanga (spirituality) to be less mysterious. I'm a people person. I believe there is power in knowledge and that power should be shared. I have more than one culture flowing in my veins, and I want both cultures to be knowledgeable about each other.

In the old days these matters were kept secret. There were good reasons for this. Sometimes such knowledge could be taken by others and used against us. For example, our Māori language was translated and written down, and before long there were Pākehā professors teaching Māori how to speak Māori, and native speakers of the reo (language) were deemed unqualified to teach it to our own people because we didn't have suitable qualifications.

However, there are also more sinister reasons why such knowledge has been kept secret. In terms of the spiritual side, over the years many people have misused wairua—they may have used it to intimidate others or even for purposes of extortion. As a result many people ended up suffering.

I want this knowledge to be used for healing. I want people to understand about wairua so that they are not left in the dark and intimidated by it. I want them to have the knowledge and tools to become part and parcel of it. I want people to be participants rather than merely spectators. I hope you will appreciate how this has worked out for young people like George in Chapter 4 and Tangi in Chapter 7.

Mauri, Mana, and Tapu

Understanding these three concepts can help families make sense of wairuatanga. I have my own way of explaining mauri, mana, and tapu which you can read about in other chapters, for example, in my first session with Tangi in Chapter 7. The concepts are not easy to translate because they are relational terms and there are no English words that capture their essence.

A person's *mauri* is often described as their 'life force'. Even objects can have a mauri. But even more than this, mauri as it has been taught to me is about being in relationship to Te Kaihanga (the creator), who is the life force. Mauri is our connection to Te Kaihanga.

I view *tapu* as the sacredness of that relationship. Tapu also refers to the state of something that is sacred or forbidden, such as a person, a place, or even an object or ritual.

These concepts are illustrated well in Chapter 5 in Caleb's story: mauri helps us understand how his unusual experiences came about, and understanding tapu helps us understand why those experiences happened in the first place. Caleb unknowingly breached a tapu, and as you read that story you will see that is one of the big learnings for him.

Mana is the spiritual authority, energy, or power embodied in a person or whānau (family) that comes from their relationship with Te Kaihanga and other key relationships. It gives them the authority to have control over themselves, their circumstances, and other entities that may be impinging on them. This is very important for people who are having unusual experiences that are spiritual but might be misdiagnosed as psychosis, such as hearing a voice or seeing something others can't see. You will read about this in action with most of the stories that follow, particularly George in Chapter 4 and Tangi in Chapter 7. For these young people, gaining understanding about mana was necessary for their healing and reclaiming their well-being.

However, even though mana is about having authority over your space, it's not about domination of others. It's about having control over your own situation. It's about being in control of your own behaviour and not hurting others. I use the concept of mana in my violence prevention work. Mana is about honour, it's about your values and beliefs. It is also about protection. So if you are taking care of the mana of your family, then you are protecting them from harm, keeping them safe, and showing them respect.

Those of you who are unfamiliar with these three concepts may find them mysterious. In the coming chapters, however, you will see how they can be applied practically in your life, and how the remarkable young people we worked with made use of such ideas to take charge of their own lives.

Wairua and Christianity

In early 2005, I was employed as the cultural therapist at Te Whare Mārie, which is the name of the Māori mental health service in Porirua, near Wellington. It was here that I first met Allister. For me, starting work at Te Whare Mārie was significant because it was a Māori service. When I was young, my kuia often told me to learn the Pākehā ways so I could get a good job. I wish she was still alive to see me being paid to be Māori!

Even though it was a Māori service, run on a marae (meeting house), and had good cultural practices, there was limited knowledge about wairua in the team at that time. Naturally enough, for some people, wairua is all about their Christian faith. I don't have a problem with that. For me, Io (God) is my source—I can do nothing without that. Anything useful, any healing, can only come from that source. It's not me doing it. And the good thing about people who come to wairua from a Christian point of view is that most of them come in a way of love. And God is portrayed as love. I think this can be very healing. You can read about the healing power of a grandmother's love in Shannon's story in Chapter 3 and a mother's love in Chapter 4.

There is a waiata (song) that says: 'Whakarongo ki te reo, e pupū ake nei. Ko te reo aroha.' It means, 'Listen to the voice that bubbles forth. It is the voice of love.' For me, the voice of love is no different from the voice of God.

However, there are limitations to this viewpoint. Christianity got very tied up in colonisation. The Bible was used to dispossess us of a lot of land—in that way it was misused and even abused. And in more subtle ways Christianity dispossessed us of some of our old understandings about wairua. For example, anything unseen that isn't understood often gets labelled as demonic, and that's not helpful. I don't go along with the idea that the Christian way is the only way. If the spiritual destination is the same, then it doesn't matter how we get there as long as we are all moving in the same direction. If I was going along in a beat-up old Holden, and someone else had a limousine, and someone else was on a Yamaha, it doesn't matter as long as the goal is the same. It's about respecting one another, no matter what vehicle you happen to be travelling in.

I often refer to Io as God. Io consists of two sounds: the 'I' is the essence, and the 'o' is the enormity of that essence. Reverend Māori Marsden (Royal, 2003) described Io this way:

> All existent being derives from a common centre. Everything depends for its existence, whether in this world, or in that behind it, upon mauri (life-force) which originates in Io-take-take (Io-the-first-cause). Io, whose mauri is primary and whose mauri both unifies all things and at the same time bestows them with unique qualities, provides for unity in diversity. Man is therefore an integral part both of the natural and spiritual order, for mauri animates all things. From this basic conviction derives the holistic approach of the Māori to all life.
>
> *(p. 95)*

For me, there is no difference between Io, the Christian God, or any other version of God.

When you read the stories you will notice that I make use of biblical references in my mahi. In fact, I've never read the Bible, but many of our whānau have been influenced by Christianity. I use those references so that people might find the wairua concepts easier to relate to. We've been doing this for a long time. Te Kooti used psalms from the Old Testament in his teachings, and the prophets Wiremu Rātana and Rua Kēnana often referred to the Bible in their kōrero.

Early Guidance

My kuia Te Awhimate guided me in my life in so many ways. She was recognised as a matekite (seer of sickness or death) and became known in our whānau for her healing practice. Many times I witnessed her doing mahi wairua (spiritual healing work). My earliest memory goes back to when I was three years old. I remember I would wake in the early hours of the morning. I would get up out of bed. I felt like I was being led towards the door of our whare (house). I can clearly recall seeing the door handle that was too high for me to reach turning and opening of its own accord. I would walk out of the whare and into the paddock. At that point I would hear my Nanny yelling out to me, 'E Wire, kia tūpato!' (Wiremu, be careful!). Her cry would snap me out of it. Afterwards Nanny would reassure me, 'We need to look after you, we need to be careful with you!' and she would tell me stories of people who had certain gifts who had been 'taken'. Because of their gifts, she believed that they had been vulnerable to tūrehu (spirit creatures).

Many of the principles I use in my mahi today came from her influence. For example, I'm always looking for an opportunity to whakamana (strengthen the mana of) a young person or whānau that I'm working with. I first saw this with my Nan, who always made sure to enhance the mana of those around her. She was herself a very humble person. I later learned the hard way that I had to be vigilant about this in my mahi for my own spiritual well-being. She had a saying, 'Me whakaiti koe i a koe, mā ētahi koe e whakanui', which meant: 'You must always be the least, and let others raise you up.' That was a whakatauākī (proverb) that she not only instilled in us but expected us to live by. It was permissible for others to praise our whānau, but we were not to put ourselves up. We were to be the least of the least.

My Nanny was also very careful about the power of words. I remember her telling me as a teenager, 'Because of the gift you have, you must never speak ill of anybody, even in anger. Do not swear at anybody. If you do, you could do them harm.' I learned to be very careful about what I said to people, especially if I got angry.

There was another form of protection that my Nanny insisted that I live by. She believed that spiritual dis-ease could result from unresolved conflict, or raruraru, between people. Her philosophy was 'Utua te kino ki te pai', which means 'bless or do good to those who would curse or harm you'. She insisted any disagreement be resolved promptly: my Nanny lived by the saying that you should never let the sun go down on your anger. These are just a few of the many healing principles she passed down to me.

Our whānau spoke only te reo Māori (Māori language) and so, because I suddenly had to speak English for the first time, starting primary school in Tiniroto was a real shock for me. I left school when I was 13, and over the years since then I've worked in many roles. I was a shearer, a fencer, and a scrubcutter. Later I worked as a musician and a songwriter. I was also a Māori activist and youth worker. As a teenager I got involved in the gangs and ended up in jail for a time. Those experiences instilled in me a real passion for youth work. After working with youth at risk for a long time, I joined the crisis mental health team at Gisborne Hospital as a cultural worker in the late 1990s.

Working Together

Allister and I were on the same team at Te Whare Mārie for about two or three years before we started to meet families together. Maybe we needed that time to suss each other out. I could see that he had few peers when it came to the clinical side. But he approached things differently from other doctors I'd worked with—almost in a Māori way. Ngāwari is a word that means going with the flow, a considerate, peaceful manner. Allister would think of the things that could be peaceful first, rather than criticising someone: he would look for a solution before going into it gung ho and knocking all the walls down. Another thing that caught my attention was his openness about spirituality. I could tell he was already on his own journey there. Despite his obvious clinical knowledge, I noticed that he was prepared to explore an avenue other than one he was familiar with. He wasn't just saying, 'This is a clinical thing and I have all the answers.' If people were in any way concerned about where they were with the cultural side of their experience, he would say, 'Well, I know someone who might know something about this. Would you like to meet with him?'

After a while Allister and I got to talking about a young person we were meeting with together. That was Caleb, who you will read about in Chapter 5. Allister asked me all sorts of questions about how to understand Caleb's situation. Later, with Caleb's permission, we presented a talk to the local psychiatrists' group about what happened to him—the doctors were interested. And some time later, after we had been meeting other families together, I suggested to Allister that we could write a book about our work together. Even though I left Te Whare Mārie in 2010, Allister continued to consult me about young people and families with wairua problems, and we usually collaborated on this mahi.

Some people might wonder why I would want to work with a Pākehā psychiatrist. Funnily enough, I did tell Allister early on that I didn't trust Pākehās—but I knew I could make that statement because I felt comfortable about doing that with him. He probably thought about it and had reached a very similar conclusion: 'I don't trust you blimmin' Māoris either!' We have now been working together for about 10 years, and each time we work together increases our trust in one another.

Tātaihono

There is a saying, 'Āpiti hono, tātai hono.' Hono means to join, and this saying means, 'Let that which has been joined remain intact.' Tātaihono can be about reparation, reconciliation, collaboration, and connection. It is about a binding together, a kind of spiritual binding that gives unity and strength. Often at the end of a tangi (bereavement ritual), this whakatauākī will be referred to. In that context it can mean, 'Let the dead be with the dead and the living be with the living', which is about maintaining the spiritual safety of the living.

Tātaihono is an active process. In our case it is about collaborating between our Māori and Pākehā points of view. We both have to put the effort in. It requires a commitment and a genuine relationship. Sometimes it's as if you are on a steep incline and you have to hold fast to your footing; otherwise, you could slip off. There is that history of colonisation in there. For that reason we had to find a way to reconcile and forgive those things that have taken place between our cultures. At the same time there is manaakitanga, giving mana to another person. Giving mana is for me the basis of our mutual respect. Another thing that binds us together is our love of people.

Allister

When I first met Wiremu, I had just completed my training as a child and adolescent psychiatrist and had returned home to New Zealand and begun working at Te Whare Mārie in Porirua. As a recently qualified professional, I was very earnestly focused on doing my job as a child and adolescent psychiatrist and not paying much heed to different points of view about wairua.

I have to admit Wiremu made an immediate impression on me. One day early on, the small work car I was using had a flat tyre. When I discovered the jack was missing, Wiremu offered his assistance. I was taken aback when he reached down and proceeded to lift the front of the car up by the bumper! He would often help me with Māori language and gave me karakia (prayers) to learn. Kindness permeated his interactions with everyone. He encouraged me to learn the guitar by telling me, 'Well, you only need to learn three chords and you can play almost anything.' For me this illustrates his approach to teaching and therapy—he is always encouraging, and he finds ways to explain complex things in a simple way so that they seem possible and achievable. So I learned to play the guitar.

Despite his warmth, during the first two years we were colleagues, I had little idea about what he did as a cultural therapist. During our multidisciplinary team meetings, Wiremu hardly said anything. Still, I sensed he was quietly observing what was going on. Some time later, I heard a couple of our clinicians talking about Wiremu meeting with families with extremely complex problems: they described surprisingly positive outcomes. That got my attention. However, whenever I approached Wiremu to discuss this, he played it down with his customary humility.

When Caleb (see Chapter 5) came to our service, I was curious about this young person's remarkable experience. Wiremu sat down with me and patiently answered my numerous questions. He had a knack for explaining complicated cultural concepts in a way I could grasp. After this, I asked him if I could sit in the next time he was seeing a family I had referred to him.

Later chapters tell stories of a very few of the young people and families we have met together. Each of these stories illustrates a situation in which Wiremu's intervention made a positive impact on the young person and their family. Many of the results seemed dramatic and surprising to me. At the conclusion of the meeting with George in Chapter 4, I could see how well George and his mother had engaged with Wiremu, but I wasn't at all prepared for the transformation that George experienced subsequently. Wiremu, however, didn't seem surprised in the least. Once he was clear that there was a spiritual problem that he could address, he seemed quietly confident that there would be a positive result. I liked Wiremu's way of relating to families, but it was the clinical outcomes that influenced me most. Over time I learnt to trust his judgement and felt steadily more confident about referring young people and families to him.

Background and Influences

When David, our co-author, encouraged Wiremu and me to write about our respective background and experiences of each other, my first response was reticence. From my viewpoint Wiremu's background is likely to be much more interesting for our readers, and I considered it my job to create space for Wiremu's story to be told, as well as describing my role as a psychiatrist. But when I raised this with Wiremu, he said that it was a joint venture and if I wasn't going to write about myself, then he wouldn't either!

I grew up in Christchurch and I am Pākehā on both sides of my family. My ancestors came from Ireland and England and settled in Canterbury in the latter years of the nineteenth century. Looking back, my early life in Christchurch afforded me little exposure to Māori and Pacific cultures. Ironically, during my medical elective in London in 1990, a German child psychiatrist advised me to return home to New Zealand and acquaint myself with the Just Therapy team and David Epston. He assured me these therapists were at the forefront of some of the most interesting ideas in family therapy. I had travelled all the way around the world to be told that there were some gems on my own doorstep that I had never heard of. I resolved to find out more on my return home.

The Just Therapy team he was referring to consisted of Warihi Campbell, Taimalieutu Kiwi Tamasese, Flora Tuhaka, and Charles Waldegrave. Their Anglican Social Services agency was based at the Family Centre in Lower Hutt. They were renowned for their strong emphasis on social justice and cultural perspectives in guiding their family therapy approach (Waldegrave et al., 2003). They were one of the first agencies in Aotearoa (New Zealand) to adopt a three-tikanga (custom) structure with Māori, Samoan, and Pākehā sections, and they developed innovative practices of accountability along lines of culture and gender.

During my first year as a junior doctor, I attended a training course at the Family Centre and was moved by the way they were grappling with some of the most difficult problems facing the families they encountered. Their outspoken approach to social inequities led them to join homeless families protesting at the local government housing agency. They were at the forefront of poverty action groups. I found myself drawn to the strong spiritual values forming the foundation of their approach, which resonated with the values in the community in which I had grown up in Christchurch. But the greatest influences on my developing understandings were the stories from the Māori and Samoan workers about their work with Māori and Samoan families.

The next year I was a participant in one of David Epston's workshops in Auckland. David, now well known as one of the founders of narrative therapy, has remained a strong influence on my thinking and practice ever since. This mentoring relationship has endured over the last 20 years. It was due to this relationship of respect and trust and his skill as a writer that Wiremu and I asked David to join us as a co-author on this book. We turn now to David for his perspective.

David

This longstanding partnership between a Māori healer and a psychiatrist in good standing intrigued me, especially as I had known and mentored Allister since he was a junior doctor with a burning passion to extend the reach of his 'healing' beyond the usual bounds of biomedicine. I followed him through his psychiatry training here in New Zealand and later his child psychiatry specialisation in Melbourne. On his return to New Zealand, it was no surprise to me that he was appointed to Te Whare Mārie and Health Pasifika, two of the first dedicated Māori and Pacific child and adolescent mental health services in New Zealand.

He joined a supervision group I ran in Wellington over the next five years, and it was here that my colleagues and I would hear of this project. We could not disguise our avid interest. When we learned that Wiremu had requested that Allister assist him to write up his practice, we all supported him in principle to do so. Allister then approached me for my assistance to create a 'style', along the lines of 'case stories'—a form that most of my publications had taken. I happily agreed to join Wiremu and Allister in such an undertaking, knowing that we would have to lay down the track ahead of us rather than appeal to some extant 'genre'. This proverbial track was laid in the give and take between us all. Each story grew by lamination as each draft came and went between our respective computers. Over time, having read across the transcultural psychiatry literature and consulted colleagues in this field, I realised that this book might do something not ever done before to my knowledge. First of all, the sessions had been prudently recorded and transcribed: the outcomes could be scrupulously reviewed with up to six year-long follow-ups. Allister's practice could be refereed by senior psychiatric colleagues. And most importantly, the two sides—Wiremu's and Allister's versions of events standing side by side—could now be easily submitted to and reviewed by third parties, especially by the patients concerned and their families. And for me, I could sit and watch as well as learn as Wiremu and Allister consolidated their bicultural and biprofessional partnership. That was surely a joy to behold.

Allister

The year I met David, I arranged for a year-long placement at the Family Centre. I was motivated to learn more about the Just Therapy approach to family therapy. However, the experiences that had the most impact on me were not the ones I was expecting. I recall an enlightening visit to the supermarket with a client from the Family Centre, a Māori woman in her late fifties with severe asthma. As a sickness beneficiary, she impressed me with her knowledge of the relative prices of all the basic grocery items and explained to me the basic food items she was regularly unable to afford when unexpected costs such as medical expenses cropped up. Having come from a middle-class background, where my material needs had always been provided for, this awakened me to the impact of poverty on her life and the lives of many other families.

Because of the Family Centre's strong local relationships, I found myself face to face with Māori community life. It wasn't long before I attended a tangi for the first time. This experience of communal Māori expressions of grief and loss seemed qualitatively different from those of the culture I had grown up in. We were regular visitors to a local marae in Wainuiomata. I attended the Family Therapy conference with the team, and I have vivid memories of staying on a marae in the settlement of Rūātoki, with the morning mists shrouding the surrounding hills, in the heart of Tūhoe country. During this time I heard stories of the impact of colonisation in New Zealand that I had never been taught in my Pākehā schooling. I talked to people who had been land rights protesters at Bastion Point in the late 1970s. They told me a totally different story than the one I had gleaned as a child from the mainstream media coverage of those events.

One of my greatest learning experiences that year was seeing the way the Family Centre team members worked together. I noticed that the Pākehā team members had a very strong commitment to the cultural values of their Māori and Samoan colleagues. Although there were robust discussions at times, I saw how they enacted their values of gender equality and cultural accountability in their work together (Waldegrave et al., 2003). This was a model for me of how a strong and cohesive relationship between Pākehā and Māori, or between Pālagi and Samoan, colleagues could contribute significantly, at a time in our history when other radical voices would have opposed a Pākehā role in Māori matters.

I learned that the heart of the Family Centre cohesion and commitment to each other came from their individual and collective spirituality, exemplified by the cultural and spiritual practices that the team adhered to. They exhibited a broad acceptance of different spiritual points of view, and especially Māori and Pacific traditions. I heard the story of Warihi Campbell's intervention with two young Māori men in jail who both appeared tormented by some unseen influence. The psychiatrist was concerned about sudden-onset psychosis; however, their distress was abruptly relieved when Warihi visited their cell and sprinkled holy water around it while reciting a karakia (Waldegrave et al., 2003).

The next year I worked in paediatrics and then commenced my training in psychiatry, during which I was fortunate to work with a number of very skilled and compassionate psychiatrists. After five years of general training in psychiatry, I specialised in child and adolescent psychiatry in Lower Hutt and later in Melbourne. From time to time my curiosity was aroused by meeting with young people who shared experiences that seemed hard to account for using traditional psychiatric paradigms.

Two years after my return to New Zealand I was asked to see Tane, a 14-year-old Samoan boy who had been admitted to the children's ward at our local hospital. His family had become very concerned about his sudden onset of uncharacteristically withdrawn behaviour. They recounted several situations in which he appeared not to recognise someone well known to him. The trainee psychiatrist who was asked to see him for an assessment recorded 'auditory hallucinations' and 'visual hallucinations' of his deceased grandfather. Tane was given a thorough physical examination to look for a possible brain problem to account for these symptoms. His blood tests and computed tomography (CT) head scan were all normal, but after a couple of days in hospital he discharged himself and refused to return for the brain wave recording (electroencephalogram, or EEG) that had been arranged.

Although Tane decided not to meet with me, I met his mother at home. She said that Tane had been very close to his grandfather, who had died six months before. Prior to this he had been conscientious in attending school and participating in his studies. Over subsequent months his behaviour changed. He took to truanting and hanging out with peers who were using illicit drugs. By the time he left hospital, he had explained to his mother what was going on. In the preceding days his deceased grandfather had appeared before him on several occasions. At first he was alarmed by this. He was especially perturbed when his grandfather gave him a good telling off for skipping class and smoking dope with his friends, insisting in no uncertain terms that he return to school immediately. Once she heard this explanation, his mother was reassured about her son's state of mind. She didn't insist that he return to hospital for the final tests. She was now convinced that this was a spiritual experience and therefore a normal phenomenon from a Samoan point of view. Over the ensuing weeks, her son reported seeing his grandfather on further occasions and receiving messages from him. He reverted to his previous studious habits and stopped accompanying his errant peers. He relayed to his mother that his grandfather had expressed satisfaction with the preparations for the unveiling later in the year and was pleased that the family were all getting together for a wedding. Tane's cousins were said to be jealous that Tane had been chosen by the grandfather for these special visitations. His mother assured me that Tane was very happy that his grandfather was still in his life and was opposed to any intervention that might reduce or remove these experiences.

Here we had a young person who had been getting into trouble after his grandfather's death. He reported the sudden onset of vivid visual and auditory experiences. His sudden change in behaviour suggested that the experiences were so compelling that they were unlikely to be accounted for by imagination or fantasy. The figure he saw not only looked like his grandfather and sounded like his grandfather, but behaved in a way that was consistent with his relationship with his grandfather when he was alive. Not only that, but Tane's experience led him to desist from the behaviours that were becoming a concern for his family.

A psychiatric disorder is defined in part by the degree of impairment and lack of well-being in someone's life, but this situation had the opposite effect. The appearance of his deceased grandfather in his life, once he had adjusted to it in the first few days, was quite clearly life enhancing, resulting in greater well-being. In addition, the usual diagnostic classification systems require us to consider the views of others from the same cultural group before concluding that an experience might be pathological. Neither Tane's mother nor my Samoan colleagues thought that Tane's experience was a problem. They were clear that it was consistent with what was commonly accepted in Samoan culture.

Tane's situation intrigued me. My Samoan colleagues explained that Samoan culture generally accepts that deceased ancestors have a number of ways of communicating with the living, and these interactions are often considered supportive and comforting. In fa'asamoa (the Samoan worldview) a person's spirit can continue to exist after the death of their body, and thus this experience could be explained by the presence of that spirit. From this point of view then, if Tane's grandfather had been present in spirit at the time when Tane saw him, then the term 'hallucination', which describes a perception in the absence of any external stimulus, is inadequate, unhelpful, and misleading. In psychiatry we don't have language to describe such an experience. If we don't have language, then such experiences are likely to go undescribed. In addition, we are trained to categorise human experience in certain ways, and thus phenomena that fall outside the usual categories of experience are easy to dismiss or misinterpret. We focus on the patterns we recognise and often dismiss the exceptions. We may notice them. They may briefly hold our interest, but then they quickly drop out of our awareness because we haven't been able to make sense of them. But the spirit of enquiry that is at the heart of scientific endeavour invites us to examine the exceptions more closely and to arrive at ways of describing and understanding them. If we are serious about expanding our understanding of the overlapping zones between psychiatry and culture, then it is exactly these exceptional experiences to which we should be attending.

Our purpose in this book is to do that—to attend to such experiences and take them seriously. In subsequent chapters we will tell the stories of five young people and their unique experiences in these overlapping zones. Each of these young people and some of their family members have consented to having their stories told and have offered their own accounts of their experiences of Wiremu's healing work.

We will describe in detail their involvement in our mental health services. Care has been taken to describe their presenting problems in enough detail that readers who are mental health clinicians will be able to come to their own conclusions about our interpretations and conclusions. In addition, we have asked for review from our advisory panel of senior psychiatrists to ensure that each chapter reaches conclusions that are supported by our psychiatrist peers. Our goal is to make these healing stories accessible to a wide readership. We have deliberately written in a style that can be understood by nonprofessional readers. In each story we reflect on the meaning of what happened from at least three perspectives: that of the psychiatrist, that of the Māori healer, and that of the young person and their family. In these reflections, we have chosen to give greater emphasis to perspectives that are less often articulated and given attention: those of Wiremu and the young people, whose courage to share their stories has enriched our understanding and challenged traditional conceptions of mental health. If you wish to begin with these stories, please turn to Chapter 3.

In Chapter 2 we examine in detail the cultural, historical and social context to this joining of Māori healing and psychiatrist perspectives and practices at this time in Aotearoa (New Zealand).

Notes

1. My understanding of matekite and matakite was passed down to me by my kuia. To me, matekite is the ability to see sickness in people, or something in the wairua that may be disturbing them, or see people who have already passed on. The purpose of the insight that matekite gives me is so I can offer help. Matakite is generally used to describe the ability to see beyond the here and now. But for me, it refers to foresight, the ability to see something before it happens. Often these abilities go together.
2. *Diagnostic and Statistical Manual of Mental Disorders*, published by the American Psychiatric Association and often used by mental health clinicians as a guide to diagnosis. The latest iteration of this manual, the DSM-5, was published in May 2013.

References

American Psychiatric Association. (2013) *Diagnostic and statistical manual of mental disorders*, DSM-5 (5th edn). American Psychiatric Association, Arlington.

Royal, T.A.C. (ed.) (2003) *The woven universe: Selected writings of Rev. Māori Marsden*. The Estate of Rev. Māori Marsden, Ōtaki.

Waldegrave, C., Tamasese, K., Tuhaka, F. & Campbell, W. (2003) *Just Therapy- a journey: A collection of papers from the Just Therapy Team, New Zealand*. Dulwich Centre Publications, Adelaide.

2

CONTEXT

Wiremu

According to an ancient karakia, Tānenuiārangi ascended to the heavenly realms, where he obtained the three kete (baskets) of knowledge. This may sound like he flew up to heaven wearing a superman suit. But to me, he was on an internal hīkoi (journey). These kete contain knowledge of the natural world around us, but also knowledge of that beyond what we can see. So he was on a quest, primarily a spiritual one. You could say he was a kind of spiritual researcher. And he brought back this knowledge with him to help us know how we could live as human beings.

So Tānenuiārangi brought the three baskets back and planted them into mother earth, who we call Papatūānuku. And not only did he plant them, but he tamped them and he moulded them, and out of that came us as humans. So for me, if I go back far enough in my whakapapa (genealogy) then I came out of Papatūānuku. So I have that relationship to her. I also have my relationship to Ranginui (our sky father), because I'm dependent on the sun for things to grow. I'm dependent on that water to fall from the heavens to sustain, revitalise, and purify us. Also, I have an unseen but felt relationship with Te Kaihanga, with the creator, who is my source.

Spirituality is woven into my relationship with the land. My well-being cannot be separated from that. So I would say that holistic healing has to include our relationships to our environment. And this affinity with Papatūānuku is reflected in our worldview in many other ways. When a child is born and their pito (umbilical cord) is severed, the whenua (placenta) is separated from the baby. And so we say, 'Mai te whenua ki te whenua', which means literally 'from the earth to the earth'. The placenta is deemed to be part of the earth. From that birthing process, the whenua, which provided all the nourishment for that baby in the womb, is given back to the earth. Thus we have this belief that we come from the earth. It all started from that time when those kete of knowledge were planted. After the placenta has been given back to the earth, we believe that the responsibility for our well-being goes to Papatūānuku who gives us sustenance during the course of our life.

Being Indigenous

For me, being indigenous is about my connection to the land. Not only do I come from the land, but my identity is intimately bound to my places of belonging. So as Māori, when we talk about who we are, we talk about our mountains, our rivers, and our ancestral lands. As you can see from the story of Tānenuiārangi, we are connected to Papatūānuku, and we are especially tied to the whenua, or land where our pito is buried.

Indigenous Knowledge

This chapter is about the knowledge that we need to do this mahi (work). It is about indigenous knowledge and other kinds of knowledge. The story of Tānenuiārangi is an example of indigenous knowledge. It has been handed down to us from our ancestors. It helps us make sense of our experience and the world around us.

One of the biggest differences for me between indigenous knowledge and Western scientific knowledge is that indigenous knowledge takes account of spirituality. And so I often say:

> I hangaia tātou e te kaihanga, kia hīkoi tātou te hīkoi tāngata.
>
> 'We were created by Io (God) to journey this earth as humans. First and foremost we are spiritual beings experiencing a human existence.'

I use this whakatauākī (proverb) to explain my experience that wairua (spirituality) is the foundation for everything else in life. In terms of theory, for me there is nothing more basic than this.

There are many knowledge baskets that we might draw from to explain our mahi together. Because our mahi is a lot about wairua, I have plenty to say about spirituality in later chapters. But there is history and the impacts of colonisation on us as Māori that are important to understand too. And as Allister will outline, many other indigenous peoples have been similarly affected.

Allister

On the first day I visited the Family Centre, I noticed a small poster on the wall beside a table laden with soup, bread rolls, seafood and salad for our shared meal at lunchtime. After Warihi Campbell had blessed the food for all of us, my eye was drawn again to the message on the poster:

> Washing one's hands of the conflict between the powerful and the powerless means to side with the powerful, not to be neutral.

This statement from Paulo Freire (1985) got me reflecting on some of the challenging ideas that the Just Therapy team had been leading us through that morning. After the pōwhiri (welcome), Flora Tuhaka, Warihi Campbell, Taimalieutu Kiwi Tamasese, and Charles Waldegrave had touched on historical events in Aotearoa that had critically shaped relationships between Māori and Pākehā, as well as between Pākehā (or Pālagi) and our Samoan and other Pacific neighbours. They argued that it is not possible to attend to these relationships without an awareness of the historical context. In particular, they suggested that the Māori and Pacific versions of history have often been silenced and remain unknown to many Pākehā New Zealanders.

Charles then talked about traditions of Western thinking that had contributed to the development of modern-day social sciences, psychology and psychiatry, and the therapeutic practices associated with those disciplines. He explained that positivism, the view that knowledge can only come from scientific verification, had been challenged in the European world by postmodern thinking. When an event happens in the physical world, a positivist approach would try to find an objective or scientific explanation to explain what happened. Postmodernism tells us that there is no such thing as an objective explanation. People give meaning to events according to beliefs they have, shaped by the cultures they come from. The values of these cultures have been moulded by interactions over generations.

However, Charles went on, this postmodernist position can be criticised because it seems to be suggesting that all explanations are of equal value. The problem with this approach can be seen most clearly in cases of manifest injustice. Victims or survivors of abuse would offer distinctly different meanings to the physical events of the abuse than would most perpetrators. Therefore, proponents of critical postmodernism have responded to this dilemma by talking about preferred meanings, derived from particular values. For example, Charles continued, gender equity may be considered preferable to male control, or cultural self-determination may be valued preferentially over the domination of one culture by another (Waldegrave, 2012). The question of values is central to this philosophical position.

Charles's explanation of the critical postmodern position made sense to me. It also got me thinking back on my medical school experiences and learning. Although we had some excellent teachers, little attention was given to the philosophical underpinnings of the scientific paradigms we were being initiated into. On reflection, I could see that I had been left with an impression that science offered a window into some universal truth. Charles's argument freed me from a scientific monopoly on what is known and what could be known. It left me with the intellectual space for the consideration of other worldviews. However, Charles went on to point out that whereas postmodern thinking offered a European, philosophical critique of the monopoly of positivist thinking, in fact there were many other challenges to positivism, especially from Māori, Pacific, and other indigenous viewpoints. This tradition of Western thought, albeit powerful, was just as much an outcome of culture as any other.

At this point Taimalieutu Kiwi Tamasese spoke. She said that from her position as a Samoan woman, Eurocentric knowledge such as scientific rationality had been integral to colonisation of Pacific peoples. She explained that the philosophical teachings of European men such as Descartes may have ushered in the age of reason from a European point of view, but from a Samoan point of view they made no sense. From a Samoan point of view, a person's sense of identity was tied up with a collective perspective rather than an individual mind (Tamasese et al., 2005). To quote Tui Atua Tupua Tamasese (2009):

> . . . we, as Samoans, Pacific or Maori peoples, are not individuals; we are integral parts of the cosmos. We share a divinity with our ancestors—the land, the seas and the skies. We are not individuals because we share a *tofi* (inheritance) with our families, our villages and our nations. We belong to our families and our families belong to us. We belong to our villages and our villages belong to us. We belong to our nation and our nation belongs to us. This is the essence of our sense of Maori and Pacific belonging.
>
> *(p. 212)*

Taimalie went on to explain that from indigenous Samoan and Māori perspectives, identity is much more connected to a collective sense of self than an individual sense of self. Furthermore, spirituality is at the heart of these indigenous worldviews, whereas Western perspectives are likely to be secular. Whereas Western traditions in the spirit of Cartesian dualism tend to look at things in terms of their component parts so that people can be separated into a mind and a body, indigenous perspectives tend to be holistic. Indigenous worldviews tend to have an ecological focus, whereas the worldviews that Western cultures foisted on indigenous communities in many parts of the world through processes of colonisation have been overwhelmingly materialistic and individualistic.

Taimalie pointed out that the more obvious devastation of colonisation historically often involved murder, the forced removal of land, and the introduction of diseases. However, the more insidious and ultimately more damaging effects were from making a people and their language disappear through other means. Western trained health professionals and therapists could easily contribute to perpetrating colonisation processes with indigenous clients if the therapies they were offering were secular; individually focused; and ignored the context of their language, identity and culture, places of belonging, and the difficulties in their lives such as poverty, abuses of power, and other forms of injustice (Tamasese, 2012).

I felt challenged and moved by the compelling logic of the case that the Just Therapy team had made: colonisation is alive and well and thriving in most modern clinic and therapeutic settings where indigenous people may be seen. But even more unsettling was Freire's assertion that maintaining my comfortable neutrality was an unsatisfactory response. The temptation to shrug my shoulders and put this problem in the 'too hard' basket was quite strong. After all, what could I do as an individual to remedy such a pervasive and extensive historical problem? Despite this feeling of helplessness, I was curious to find out more about the history of Māori and Pākehā relationships that I had only been partially aware of in my school years.

Indigenous People in Aotearoa (New Zealand)

Māori are of Polynesian descent and arrived in Aotearoa (New Zealand) during a time of great Polynesian voyaging across the Pacific at least 1000 years ago (Belich, 1996; Durie, 2011; King, 2003; Walker, 1990). Over ensuing generations before the arrival of the first British settlers 200 years ago, Māori evolved a distinctive language and culture suited to the temperate conditions of their environment (Durie, 2011; Walker, 1990). Before European contact, Māori identity was focused on iwi, or tribal affiliations; however, with the appearance of white strangers on their shores, according to Ranginui Walker (1990), Māori chose the word pākehā to describe the strange pale look of these newcomers, while referring to themselves as māori (normal or natural).

Wiremu tells of the following prophecy:

> About 250 years ago, before Captain Cook first visited these shores, a prophet called Toiroa Ikariki from Nukutauroa on Māhia Peninsula made a prediction. He talked about the arrival of people he called 'pakerewha'. The pakerewha referred to people who came from far away and carried a certain illness. He predicted that they would bring with them a God, 'he whose son was murdered'. Toiroa predicted that this God would be a good God, but there would still be dark times. So he was prophesying that Christianity would come to these shores. Of course, the illness he was referring to could have been small pox or influenza or other illnesses that the Pākehā later brought with them that knocked many of us over in those years.

By 1840, officials on behalf of the British Crown, seeking to secure British interests in New Zealand against the threat of competing French colonial interest, and responding to Māori and other settler concerns about lawless Pākehā behaviour, drafted a treaty in English to present to a large gathering of Māori chiefs at the settlement of Waitangi for their approval (Orange, 1992). It was hastily translated into te reo Māori the night before by established Pākehā residents—and there were some key differences between the two versions. In the Māori text, the chiefs gave the Crown kāwanatanga (governance) over their land. However, their tino rangatiratanga (unqualified authority) over their land, resources, and taonga (ancestral and cultural treasures) was protected. Full rights of British citizenship were guaranteed along with a promise that Māori peoples would be protected by the Crown. In the English text, Māori were ceding their 'sovereignty'. If it had been explained to them what sovereignty meant from a British point of view, it's highly unlikely any of the chiefs present would have agreed to sign the treaty. Eventually over 500 chiefs in both the North and South islands signed the Māori version known as Te Tiriti o Waitangi (the Treaty of Waitangi) (Orange, 1992; Walker, 1990).

The Māori population in 1800, estimated at around 200,000, had dropped significantly by 1840, but Māori still outnumbered Pākehā by about 50 to 1 (Consedine & Consedine, 2012). However, within 20 years of the treaty being signed, a huge wave of Pākehā settlers, predominantly from the British Isles, outnumbered the Māori population. The promises of the treaty were ignored, and 'land wars', with the backing of the British imperial forces, resulted in vast areas of previously Māori land being 'confiscated' and brought under Pākehā control (Belich, 1996; Walker, 1990). A great deal of remaining land was taken by means of unjust legislation. By 1900 the Māori population had fallen precipitously to just 45,000, because of deaths from war and diseases such as influenza, tuberculosis, and measles, along with the effects of poverty and demoralisation associated with dispossession of land and other resources (Durie, 2011). At this time, there were widespread Pākehā predictions that Māori were heading toward extinction (Walker, 1990).

According to Wiremu:

> For us as Māori, we lost many things, but I believe the most damaging was the loss of our land. With the dispossession of our ancestral lands, our access to those spiritual ties with Papatūānuku were taken away, cutting us off from our spiritual sustenance.

For Linda Tuhiwai Smith (2012), the most significant processes of colonisation included the 'stripping away of mana' and the 'undermining of rangatiratanga', a people's right to determine their own destiny (p. 175). Māori Marsden has attested to the common patterns of colonisation of indigenous peoples, invariably comprising 'pacification' by war, law, or treaty; the seizure of lands and resources; and processes of assimilation resulting in what he termed 'cultural genocide' (Royal, 2003: p. 88).

The Impacts of Colonisation

For the indigenous reader, or others who already realise that cultural genocide is a justifiable way to describe the impacts of colonisation on indigenous peoples, the next section contains information that may be distressing and you might wish to skip it. However, it may not be obvious to all readers. I was brought up on the idea that colonisation benefited indigenous societies by introducing civilisation, roads and railways, and the benefits of modern governance systems such as democracy. To people like me, the idea of cultural genocide seemed extreme.

A range of indigenous commentators have referred to the widespread and systematic destruction of their cultures at the hands of colonial governments in these terms (Durie, 2004a; Royal, 2003; Tinker, 1993). Clearly, they are referring to a meaning that is much broader than loss of life. However, even in those terms, as with the Māori population decline through the nineteenth century, the impact of the processes and practices of colonisation on indigenous peoples in many places has been cataclysmic. In North America before the arrival of Europeans, the total population of indigenous peoples was estimated to be more than seven million: over the subsequent century or more this number fell by 90 percent (Kirmayer et al., 2009). The Iroquoian peoples, whose population was estimated at 110,000 in the early seventeenth century, had dwindled to 8000 by 1850 (Kirmayer et al., 2009). In British Columbia, the estimated Aboriginal population prior to European contact was well over 300,000 and fell by 80 percent over the subsequent 100 years (Consedine & Consedine, 2012). Disastrous epidemics, such as that of smallpox in 1862, killed one-third of the indigenous people in British Columbia at that time, but cannot account for the overall calamitous population decline.

In Australia, the notion of terra nullius, meaning literally 'empty land', was used after 1788 by colonial administrators to justify their claims on all the land in Australia, despite Aboriginal peoples having preceded them by more than 60,000 years (Durie et al., 2009). As many as 500,000 indigenous Australians were forced off land they had occupied for well over a thousand generations. Historical evidence indicates that up to 20,000 Aborigines were killed during this process (Reynolds, 1996). From a precontact population thought to be more than a million (Durie et al., 2009), by 1911, the total population of indigenous Australians was estimated to be 31,000 (Consedine & Consedine, 2012; Tatz, 1999).

In countries such as Canada, the United States, Australia, and New Zealand, a strikingly similar pattern of colonisation of indigenous communities developed (Armitage, 1995; Kunitz, 1994). In each case British colonial practices were used, which were inspired by the belief that European civilisation was genuinely superior. These practices had been honed during centuries of English rule in Ireland (Consedine & Consedine, 2012). Invariably the initial devastation to the indigenous population resulted from warfare and introduced infectious diseases. This was always followed by forced confiscation of ancestral land

and the compulsory settling of nomadic indigenous peoples. However, just as catastrophic was the active suppression of indigenous cultures, identities, languages, and forms of spiritual expression that inevitably followed. There is strong evidence that forced assimilation was carefully orchestrated (Armitage, 1995; Kunitz, 1994). In Canada, the United States, and Australia, church schooling was mandatory for indigenous children, who were forcibly removed from their families to live in boarding schools far away from their loved ones (Durie et al., 2009; Kirmayer et al., 2009; Tinker, 1993). In Canada, for over 100 years, more than 100,000 Aboriginal children were made to attend these institutions, which changed their names; degraded and suppressed their languages, cultures, and beliefs; and inculcated Anglo values and Christian theology. In the United States by the mid-1970s there were still more than 50,000 indigenous children enrolled in church schools, with the same practices designed to erode and eradicate their indigenous identities (DeJong, 1993).

In Australia, between 10 and 33 percent of Aboriginal children were forcibly removed from their families and communities between 1910 and 1970 and placed in residential schools with little or no ongoing contact with their families and communities of origin (Bringing Them Home, 1997). Recently there has been increasing evidence of the widespread physical, emotional, and sexual abuse that was perpetrated against children in these settings (Bringing Them Home, 1997; Haig-Brown, 2002; Milloy, 1999; Tinker, 1993).

Archie Fire Lame Deer, a Lakota medicine man, has given a vivid insider account of his experiences in a Catholic boarding school (Lame Deer & Erdoes, 1992). Vine Deloria (2003) has also written extensively on the destructive impact of these residential schools in the United States. In a similar vein, George Tinker (1993) wrote about the 'destruction of Indian cultures and tribal social structures' (p. 4) that resulted from such institutions and concluded that cultural genocide could be viewed as the destruction of a people by 'eroding or undermining the integrity of the culture and system of values that defines a people and gives them life' (p. 6).

In New Zealand, successive settler governments systematically suppressed Māori language, culture, and identity by banning te reo Māori in schools and excluding Māori culture and perspectives from school curricula, colonial accounts of history, and most institutions (Durie, 1998; Royal, 2003).

After World War I, New Zealand occupied Samoa, which had previously been colonised by Germany. The inept New Zealand colonial administration presided over the devastating influenza epidemic of 1918 and attempted to suppress Samoan culture. Marked dissatisfaction in the Samoan population with the administration's draconian legal measures led to the establishment of the Samoan passive resistance movement known as the Mau, whose slogan was 'Samoa mo Samoa' (Samoa for Samoans). Rising tensions by 1929 culminated in the Black Saturday incident in which New Zealand police officers shot and killed eight Mau members during a parade in Apia, including the Mau leader and high chief

Tupua Tamasese Lealofi III (Field, 1984). Although Samoa finally achieved independence in 1962, other Pacific nations, including Tokelau, Cook Islands, and Niue, have remained under New Zealand's political and colonising influence.

In Australia, between 1900 and the 1960s, mention of Aboriginal people disappeared almost entirely out of Australian history books (Reynolds, 1999). In Aotearoa (New Zealand), for decades Māori were excluded almost entirely from politics, but by 1867 they were able to vote, albeit for a third of the seats that would have been fair allocation on a per capita basis. In Canada, indigenous people were excluded from their nation's democratic process until 1967 (Kirmayer et al., 2009), and in Australia legislation was passed in the 1960s allowing Aboriginal Australians voting rights (Durie et al., 2009). In the United States, the Indian Citizenship Act of 1924 granted citizenship to Native Americans, but only if they renounced their tribal affiliations; as a result many decided not to become American citizens. In addition, many states found other ways to obstruct indigenous participation in democratic processes for decades (Deloria, 1992).

The role of women in indigenous communities has also been severely affected by colonisation. Many indigenous peoples such as those in the Pacific and North and South America had matrilineal and matriarchal traditions, which were suppressed and distorted by missionary and colonial authorities intent on reproducing the patriarchal values inherent in British and other European gender arrangements (Tamasese, 2012). In Hawai'i, Queen Lili'uokalani's reign was cut short in early 1893 by a coup led by American and European businessmen, and the queen was later imprisoned. Other examples include Haudenosaunee[1] matrilineal traditions and governing processes based on principles of balance and consensus (Hill, 2008). Tamasese (2012) has pointed out that the nuances of indigenous gender arrangements have often been lost on Western observers, who have been unable to discern the lasting effects of Christian and Western colonising influences.

Colonisation and Indigenous Healing Practices

Indigenous healing practices and beliefs were particularly targeted by colonial and missionary authorities (Deloria, 2003; Durie, 2009; Durie et al., 2009; Kirmayer et al., 2009; Tinker, 1993). In New Zealand, the Tohunga Suppression Act of 1907 banned any traditional healing activities and resulted in the disappearance of Māori healing practices, at least publicly, and loss of confidence in and access to this knowledge for many communities over the subsequent generations until the act was repealed in 1964 (Durie, 2009). In Canada, an amendment to the Indian Act in 1884 made it illegal to carry out indigenous healing ceremonies such as the 'Sun Dance' and 'Pot Latch' (Robbins & Dewar, 2011). Similarly, indigenous healing was outlawed in many parts of the United States from the late nineteenth century until the American Indian Religious Freedom Act was passed in 1978 (Deloria, 1999).

The Diversity of Indigenous Peoples

There are thought to be more than 300 million indigenous people in at least 70 countries around the world, making up as many as 5000 distinct groupings (Horton, 2006). Almost 200 million reside in countries and regions such as China, South Asia, Africa, and the former Soviet Union for which there is a distinct lack of health and socioeconomic data (Stephens et al., 2005). In Canada alone there are many indigenous languages that can be clustered into 11 major language groups (Kirmayer et al., 2009). In Australia, there were estimated to be more than 250 Aboriginal languages before European contact, and Aboriginal Australians are descended from an estimated 600 to 700 nations from across Australia, including the Torres Strait Islands (Durie et al., 2009).

According to Durie (2004b), indigenous people do not define themselves on the basis of their experience of colonisation or the social adversity and health disparities they face. However, in almost all countries where there is any data, minority indigenous communities have substantially more poverty to deal with; much higher disease and mortality rates; and markedly less access to education, health, and other resources than the general population (Stephens et al., 2005).

Indigenous Peoples and Mental Well-being

There are many challenges involved in defining mental health problems because of the wide diversity in the way people across such disparate cultural groups express distress (Kirmayer et al., 2009; Kleinman, 1980). Nonetheless there is widespread evidence that minority indigenous populations in Canada, the United States, Australia, New Zealand, and elsewhere suffer to a markedly greater degree from alcohol-related problems, youth suicide, depression, and posttraumatic conditions. They are much more likely to be diagnosed with severe mental health problems such as schizophrenia than others in the general populations of these countries (Durie et al., 2009; Kirmayer et al., 2009; MaGPIe group, 2005; Stephens et al., 2005).

In New Zealand, since the 1950s and the urbanisation of many Māori families, Māori psychiatric admission rates have risen to two to three times higher than those for Pākehā New Zealanders (Durie, 2011). Māori are more likely to present to services at a later stage and to be required to undergo compulsory treatment (Dyall, 1997). There has been a widespread perception among Māori for many years that New Zealand mental health services were not meeting their needs: their concerns included the inappropriate use of diagnoses of severe mental disorders such as schizophrenia, culturally insensitive therapies, widespread assumptions about Māori deficits, and institutional ignorance of Māori worldviews (Durie, 2011).

Māori Recovery and Development since 1900

At the time of the 2013 census in New Zealand, one in seven New Zealanders, or 598,605 people, identified with the Māori ethnic group, making up 14.9 percent of the total population, and 668,724 people were of Māori descent (Statistics New Zealand, 2013). Projections suggest that the Māori population, which has a median age of just 23.9 years, could almost double by 2051 (Pool, 1991). Alongside this remarkable population recovery, from the early years of the twentieth century there has been a steady increase in Māori participation in all areas of public life, including health, education, government, and the economy. In particular during the last two or three decades there have been major developments in the incorporation of Māori worldviews into government health policy and, subsequently, clinical practice.

Durie suggests that Māori leadership has made a major contribution to improvements in Māori health outcomes at many levels (Durie, 1998). Politicians in the early years of the twentieth century, such as Māui Pōmare and Āpirana Ngata, advocated strongly for Māori communities within the constraints of the Western monocultural government systems. Outside government, leaders such as Te Puea Hērangi worked to bring Western medical knowledge to Māori settings, such as marae in her local community (Durie, 1998; King, 1977). Despite the Tohunga Suppression Act, a few Māori healers were still influential. Tahupōtiki Wiremu Rātana attracted a large following through his healing practices based on Christian principles, and his methods were not dissimilar to other Māori healing traditions (Durie, 1998). In establishing the Rātana Church, he advocated strongly for the importance of Māori identity (Newman, 2009).

By the middle part of the century, women's organisations such as the Māori Women's Welfare League provided a strong voice for Māori community concerns, and one leader, Whina Cooper, later led 5000 people in the historic 1975 hīkoi (land rights march), walking the length of the North Island of New Zealand in protest against loss of land and to publicise a range of other Māori social and economic concerns (Durie, 1998; King, 1983). Their slogan was 'Not one more acre of Māori land to be surrendered to the Pākehā.' This public display of discontent, after many decades of exhausting legal, political, and other community avenues to effect change, heralded a shift to a form of Māori activism reminiscent of the passive resistance practices developed by Te Whiti o Rongomai and Tohu Kākahi in the Parihaka community in Taranaki 100 years before (Consedine & Consedine, 2012; Scott, 1981).

By 1977, the struggle to address land alienation intensified. Renewed Māori activism at this time was in line with indigenous protest movements in other countries. In Australia, protests such as the Aboriginal Stockmen's strike in 1946 and the Yirrkala bark petitions in 1963 were followed by Aboriginal legal action that resulted in a Royal Commission in the early 1970s and the Aboriginal Land Rights Act in 1976 (Langton & Peterson, 1983). However, the struggle to establish indigenous land rights attracted strenuous opposition from some state governments (Reynolds, 1999). In the United States, Native American protestors occupied Alcatraz Island in San Francisco Bay in 1969 and, the next year, seized the *Mayflower* during Thanksgiving Day celebrations. The American Indian Movement (AIM) takeover at Wounded Knee, South Dakota, in 1973 was followed five years later by 'the Longest Walk', when thousands of Native Americans participated in a 3200-mile protest walk across the country to bring attention to anti-Indian legislation and in support of tribal sovereignty (Deloria, 2003; Johnson et al., 1997). In Canada, First Nations and other indigenous communities have persisted with legal and other forms of protest for many years, from the Iroquois declaration of self-government at the Six Nations reserve in Brantford, Ontario, in 1959, to more recently the Oka protest in 1990 (Kirmayer et al., 2009), which led to the 1991 Royal Commission on Aboriginal Peoples. The resulting public hearings uncovered widespread abuses perpetrated in the residential school system (Kirmayer et al., 2009).

However, despite signs that some countries have begun attending to aspects of colonisation, many generations of indigenous families are still feeling the ripple effects. For clinicians and therapists meeting with an indigenous person, with or without other family members present, these effects may be difficult to discern and can easily be rendered invisible by Western psychological and psychiatric practices that focus on the individual.

Ripple Effects and Mental Health

Betty was a Māori woman in her mid-fifties when I became her doctor at Te Whare Mārie during my training in psychiatry. She was slim, and her short hair was greying beyond her years. There was something in her eyes that told me she had suffered much in the course of her life. Over the previous decade she had been admitted to hospital several times with manic symptoms, and she had also endured a number of bouts of depression that had been very distressing for her. She had been given a diagnosis of bipolar affective disorder. She tended to accept the medication she had been prescribed to stabilise her mood, but there was an air of resignation about her demeanour, as if this was yet one more indignity that she would have to bear. I gathered that she was cut off from her family of origin and had experienced considerable physical abuse by her partner. When I asked her about her earlier life, she had little to say, but hinted at family troubles with drinking. I gathered that she had become familiar with family violence as a young child—certainly her family had little money. It was at this point that I learnt that her iwi was Ngāti Whātua. She had grown up in the community at Ōkahu Bay in Auckland, before her family moved away in her primary-school years. Other members of her extended family had also suffered from mental health problems, including depression and bipolar disorder. Her adult daughter had recently been admitted to hospital with her first psychotic illness.

Reflecting on Betty's iwi affiliation, my mind turned back to the history I had heard about Ngāti Whātua and the devastating effects the loss of iwi land had on this once-thriving people.

Auckland, New Zealand's most populous city, is situated on the shores of Waitematā Harbour. Before 1840, a large area of land in the city centre was owned and inhabited as a fishing community by Ngāti Whātua. Shortly after 1840, 1200 acres had been bought for a pittance by colonial officials, who immediately subdivided it, making a huge profit (Consedine & Consedine, 2012). Collective ownership customs and Māori beliefs about sovereignty make it highly unlikely that Ngāti Whātua, as an iwi, would have agreed to permanently relinquish their ownership of this land. Numerous attempts by Ngāti Whātua leaders to address this injustice via every available legal channel over the next 135 years had been fruitless. Meanwhile, city authorities had designs on the remaining Ngāti Whātua land and made regular attempts to acquire it. In 1952, through dubious legal means, and motivated by a forthcoming visit by Queen Elizabeth, authorities burned down the ancestral village at Ōkahu Bay on the pretext of public health concerns and forcibly moved the inhabitants into nearby housing (Consedine & Consedine, 2012). They immediately took control of the land the village had stood on. Impending city council plans to subdivide this land in 1977 precipitated a 506-day occupation of the land at Takaparawhā (Bastion Point) by Māori and Pākehā protestors, culminating in one of the biggest police operations in New Zealand history: that day, 222 protestors were arrested and removed from the land under direct orders of the prime minister. The intense media attention surrounding this event ensured that Pākehā New Zealanders all over the country witnessed the disturbing scenes. The 'standard story' that Pākehā had grown up with—that New Zealand had the 'best race relations' of any country in the world—was shaken up considerably (Consedine & Consedine, 2012).

Betty

Betty recently recalled her early life at Ōkahu Bay with the following account:

My earliest memories are of playing on the beach at Ōkahu Bay, swimming and gathering sticks for the fire. Often we would go hunting for rock oysters. Other times we would clamber down the piles on the wharf and grab handfuls of baby mussels. Back up on the wharf we would open the shells and eat them just like that. We used to go picking quince and take it home for Mum to cook up into jam. I remember hopscotch and playing knuckle bones with stones. We were poor people. Our Mum used to go to second hand shops to get our clothes. But we thought that we were well dressed. Often we went to school with bare feet. But we were only children; we didn't feel the cold like old people do. The local school was mainly Pākehā. There was nothing Māori taught there. I don't know how to speak Māori. Mum used to speak it over the fence to the neighbour. She could speak Māori but she never taught us.

In 1952 the government sent in police to move us all off the land. There was a big protest. I remember this long line of police trying to force the Māoris back, all with their long black coats, and those old fashioned round hats, not like the ones they've got today. All the kids were running around. The older women were crying. The men were playing superman, trying to be strong, trying to ward off the police. It became quite ugly. People were dragged away and put in paddy wagons. It was all done because the young Queen Elizabeth was coming through and we were on the main road. Our fences were falling down and some of our houses were tin shacks. The Pākehā authorities thought it was distasteful for the Queen to be passing by such untidiness.

We couldn't stop the burning of the papa kāinga [village]. There was nothing we could do. People were devastated. That was our home for many, many years. It was our Pā (village), our marae; the urupā (burial ground) was there. Many generations had grown up there, had their children and their children's children, and died there.

After the burning of the kāinga, we were told to move into a new house up in Kitemoana Street. That's the name of the street that goes up to where the state houses are. That's where all the Māoris got booted up to. We called it 'Boot Hill'. We had no option. But Mum didn't want to go up there because it was too exposed and the sea wind would blow into the house. It was very cold. So she asked for a transfer. We got a state house in another suburb and moved away.

Allister

After I realised that Betty had grown up in Ōkahu Bay, I wondered about the possible connection between the loss of land her iwi experienced and the severe mental health problems she and other members of her whānau were facing.

In my training in psychiatry there was a strong emphasis on understanding the problems people were presenting with from biological, psychological, social, and even cultural perspectives, an approach known as the biopsychosocial model (Engel, 1980). In addition, there are social psychiatrists and child psychiatrists who focus on family systems, who give even more prominence to nonbiomedical viewpoints. Despite these voices in our profession, there remains a common tendency in psychiatry to look inside people for possible causes for mental unwellness. This way of thinking is consistent with reductionism in Western science and leads us to consider neurochemical and genetic causes as well as psychological causes internal to the individual. When other family members are affected, that is often taken as further evidence of a genetic makeup that is vulnerable to mental illness.

Mason Durie, a Māori psychiatrist and professor of Māori studies, has dubbed this way of thinking 'centripetal': it appears that some unseen force is pulling the focus of this thinking centrally, inside the person (Durie, 2009). He considers this way of thinking to be typical of psychiatry, and Western medicine in general. In contrast, for Māori and other indigenous cultures, the search for understanding of human suffering is centrifugal—that is, it flows outward from the individual to the environment and others around them. From this perspective, it makes sense to look for environmental causes that may have contributed to Betty's plight and recurrent mental health problems, not just causes internal to her. The sequence of losses inflicted on her whānau and hapū (subtribe) through loss of land, powerlessness to seek redress, unresolved outrage and grief associated with that, and the loss of mana experienced by subsequent generations are likely to be contributing factors to the circumstances of the whānau into which she was born. The effects of poverty due to loss of resources and loss of livelihood, such as markedly reduced access to traditional fishing grounds, would be relevant to understanding her predicament. And when Betty was attending her local primary school in the city in the late 1940s and early 1950s, there may well have been prejudice from local Pākehā communities uncomfortable with the Māori presence, which might have contributed to a sense of alienation and uncertainty about her identity as Māori.

Durie et al. (2009) note that in psychiatry, the strong focus on biological determinants of health and mental health has led to a range of studies into the genetic contribution to disease in indigenous populations. Although there is some evidence indicating an increased genetic risk of diabetes and kidney disease in indigenous populations, there is no evidence supporting increased genetic susceptibility to mental health conditions in indigenous peoples. Instead many commentators point to the obvious social adversity faced by these communities and the evidence that such factors are associated with higher rates of mental distress and disorder in population studies in many settings. The commentators strongly suggest that social determinants are a much more likely explanation for the widespread health and mental health disparities in indigenous populations (Durie et al., 2009; Kirmayer et al., 2009).

A survey of psychiatrists in New Zealand found that many respondents viewed low socioeconomic status as a contributing factor, and one-third believed that loss of land and colonisation could be factors in explaining why Māori are overrepresented in psychiatric institutions. However, 28 out of 212 psychiatrists surveyed believed that biological/genetic causes were at the basis of this overrepresentation. Although this was just 11 percent of the sample, all 28 were New Zealand–born and had been working in New Zealand for more than 10 years (Johnstone & Read, 2000). Given the lack of evidence to support this view that genetic vulnerability is the cause of the problem, how else can we understand the beliefs expressed by this subgroup of psychiatrists?

Tim McCreanor and Ray Nairn are Pākehā social scientists who have studied patterns in Pākehā talk about Māori over the last 30 years, using discourse analysis techniques (McCreanor, 2012; Nairn, 2012). They refer to the substance of what we say to each other as discursive resources—a linguistic inheritance derived largely from the social groups we grew up in and identify with. Pākehā have certain discursive resources that we tend to turn to when talking about Māori that have been developed and shaped over generations to help us make sense of our outsider view of what it means to be Māori. These researchers have identified more than a dozen themes of a 'standard story' that have recurred repeatedly in a range of media, political talk, and public documents over that time, which they consider indicative of entrenched negative patterns in Pākehā attitudes towards Māori (McCreanor, 2012). Such views may be shared intuitively in a Pākehā context to such an extent that when someone refers to them using certain cue words, the meaning may appear to be such obvious common sense that the speaker may feel no need to justify what they have said (Nairn, 2012).

Tim McCreanor (2012) describes the Pākehā 'standard story' portraying Māori culture as 'fundamentally inferior to that of the settlers'. Māori language, in this discourse, is viewed as irrelevant in the modern world. Māori artistic achievements don't measure up to those of European New Zealanders, and Māori cultural practices are viewed as archaic. Cue words that refer to this discourse include expressions such as 'simplistic, limited, stone-age, inefficient, inadequate, undemocratic, sexist, and phrases such as stick games, grass skirts, mud huts, five musical notes' (p. 295).

Presumably Pākehā psychiatrists who have worked in New Zealand for more than 10 years have had greater exposure to the standard discourses about 'Māori deficit' prominent in their communities and in the professional discourses about Māori than psychiatrists who have arrived or completed their training in New Zealand more recently.

Nairn highlights the importance of identifying and developing 'discursive resources' that assist Pākehā to recognise and counteract the familiar 'standard story'. For example, alternative ways of talking about Māori could acknowledge the essential role Māori culture plays in our nation's identity and character, while emphasising the value of viewing cultures as contrasting or complementing rather than better or worse than each other (McCreanor, 2012). Such views have received wider Pākehā acceptance in recent decades, as the Treaty of Waitangi has become pivotal to the debate about Māori–Pākehā relations.

Development of Indigenous Mental Health Services in New Zealand

Alongside the more public signs of Māori discontent in the 1970s and 1980s and Māori calls for the government to honour its obligations in the Treaty of Waitangi, Māori leaders in health were advocating strongly for the principles of the Treaty of Waitangi to be considered as a foundation for changes in health and other social service provisions for Māori (Durie, 1998). The Treaty of Waitangi Act, passed in 1975, cleared the way for Māori grievances pertaining to Crown breaches of the treaty to begin to be addressed (Durie, 2003). By 1984, the Waitangi Tribunal was set up to investigate Māori claims against the Crown, and shortly afterwards a Royal Commission determined that the treaty principles—those ensuring Māori partnership, participation, and protection—were relevant not only to land, forestry, and fisheries, but to all social and economic policies (Durie, 1998, 2009).

In 1985, the Department of Health recommended that the treaty be integrated into health services. By this time, the first bicultural Mental Health Unit had already been set up at Tokanui Hospital in the Waikato, which served a large Māori population. This unit offered a therapeutic blend of Māori language, customs, and values in its milieu and group programmes alongside modern psychiatric medication treatments (Durie, 1998). Te Whare Mārie, the kaupapa Māori (Māori-centred) mental health service based in Porirua, near the capital city of Wellington, was established in the early 1990s, as well as a number of bicultural units in other areas where there were large Māori populations (McCarthy, 1993). In general these units had a 'by Māori, for Māori' ethos, Māori leadership, and tended to employ Māori mental health staff and kaumātua (elders) who guided the use of Māori customs and values in their services. They fostered the development of new Māori clinicians through student placements and promoted the development of Māori therapies such as Te Tuakiri o te Ora (see Chapter 7).

Mason Durie played a key leadership role during this time, both as a psychiatrist in his work at the Oranga Hinengaro Kaupapa Māori unit in Palmerston North, and later as Professor of Māori Studies at Massey University—but also in his research and as an advisor to the Department of Health. He articulated a Māori model of health known as Te Whare Tapa Whā, synthesised from Māori views expressed by elders at many gatherings in Māori settings (Durie, 2011). In this model, four key components were compared to the walls of a house, each of which is essential to the strength and integrity of the whole. The four components were te taha wairua (spirituality), te taha whānau (family and relational values), te taha tinana (physical well-being), and te taha hinengaro (emotional and mental well-being). Durie pointed out that te taha wairua is considered by Māori to be the basis for all the other components. This model was subsequently incorporated into government frameworks and Māori models of service delivery (Durie, 1998). Elsewhere Durie had described 'three institutions' as critical to Māori health: land, language, and family (Durie, 1998).

Meanwhile other holistic Māori models were being articulated. Rangimarie Rose Pere used 'Te Wheke' (the octopus): each tentacle represented a necessary component: wairua, whānau, hinengaro, tinana, mana ake (uniqueness of individual and family), mauri (life force), hā a koro mā a kui mā (the 'breath of life' that comes from ancestors), and whatumanawa (open and healthy expression of emotion); waiora (total well-being) is represented by the eyes of the octopus (Durie, 1998; Pere, 1984; Pere, 1991). This model was also widely endorsed by Māori.

Reemergence of Indigenous Healing Practices

With renewed calls for spirituality to be attended to in Māori health, consideration was given to how Māori traditional healing practices could be incorporated into Māori health settings (Durie, 2009). Even in the 1950s several tohunga (traditional healers), such as Kapi Adams, Hori Gage, and Alec Phillips, had become well known among their Māori communities for their healing work (Durie, 1998). A 1984 survey demonstrated that 20 percent of Māori women in the sample would consult a traditional healer if they were concerned about mate Māori (illness due to a Māori cultural or spiritual problem) (Durie, 2009). There were fresh calls from Māori communities for tohunga to be included in services funded by the government, and a framework was developed for the Department of Health to contract Māori healers to work within primary care teams (Durie, 2011). Ngā Ringa Whakahaere o te Iwi Māori, a national body of Māori healers, was founded in 1993; at the request of this organisation, the Ministry of Health in 1999 released a set of standards for traditional healers, including a code of practice, standards covering responsibilities towards patients, communication with other health practitioners, and the collection and administering of rongoā (herbal medicinal preparations) (Durie, 1998, 2009).

Durie (2009) has suggested that in modern times, Māori healers may be closely aligned to their tribal areas or may be based in urban settings. He has described Māori healing processes as including three phases that attend to assessment, spiritual reparation, and the application of specific remedies for the defined problem. Assessment focuses on the presenting problem, but also on possible links with breaches of tapu[2] or relationship problems in the immediate whānau, or intergenerational problems. Remedies depend on the area of expertise of the healer, but may include mirimiri (massage), karakia (prayers or incantations), rongoā, and water- and heat-based treatments. A primary task is to restore balance between the elements of wairua, hinengaro, whānau, and tinana (Durie, 2009). This is illustrated in an account of the work of the tohunga, Hohepa Kereopa (Moon, 2003).

Indigenous Healing in Other Places

Despite the prohibitions set up by colonial governments, indigenous communities everywhere have still turned to their own healers for spiritual, physical, and psychological healing. And not only indigenous communities: the World Health Organization estimates that up to 85 percent of the world's population relies on traditional healers to meet their healthcare needs (Incayawar et al., 2009).

Indigenous community members often prefer to see a traditional healer from their own community rather than a Western practitioner; or they may choose their practitioner depending on how they perceive the nature of the problem. There is evidence that Navajo communities favour traditional healing practices, but will see a doctor who practises Western medicine for certain conditions (Kim & Kwok, 1998). A study of Native American city dwellers in Milwaukee, Wisconsin, who were affiliated with 30 different tribes, showed that 38 percent would regularly see an indigenous healer, often for problems that they perceived as spiritual, and two-thirds of those rated their healer's advice higher than their doctor's (Marbella et al., 1998). Healers included herbalists, spiritual healers, and medicine men. Sweat lodge ceremonies, spiritual healing, and herbal remedies were often used. There are a number of insider accounts of the lives of indigenous healers in North America (Crow Dog & Erdoes, 1995; Lame Deer & Erdoes, 1992; Lame Deer & Erdoes, 1972; Mohatt & Eagle Elk, 2000), South America (Kopenawa & Albert, 2013; Incayawar et al., 2009), and Africa (Somé, 1994). Other indigenous authors have drawn on traditional healing methods to address the trauma of colonisation directly in a therapeutic context (Duran, 2006). In indigenous services in Canada, such as the Six Nations Mental Health Service in the Six Nations community near Brantford, Ontario, it is widely recognised that First Nations and other indigenous peoples may well wish to pursue traditional healing, and staff will sometimes help clients access traditional healing in the local community (Wieman, 2009).

Ngangkaṟi are the Aboriginal traditional healers of the Western Desert region in Central Australia (Ngaanyatjarra Pitjantjatjara Yankunytjatjara Women's Council Aboriginal Corporation, 2013). Healers such as Rupert Langkatjukur Peter have emphasised the fundamental role of the spirit in ngangkaṟi healing:

> Everyone has a spirit. Sometimes they can lose that spirit, become dispirited, and they can become really sick. . . . We ngangkaṟi have the ability to see that situation, to assess it, to see where their spirit has gone—often it will actually leave them or be out of place. We find that spirit and place it back within people in the right place so they are balanced again and centred.
>
> *(p. 192)*

Indigenous Knowledge and Science

Although there are obvious points of difference between indigenous paradigms and Western medical approaches aligned with scientific endeavour, Durie (2004b) maintains that each worldview is not in a position to judge the other. Science and indigenous knowledge have very different principles for judging the validity of knowledge, derived from disparate philosophies and methods. Therefore, it is illogical to judge indigenous knowledge using scientific standards, just as it is unreasonable to evaluate science by the precepts of indigenous knowledge. He points out that despite the contentious nature of their relative virtues, such disputes 'distract from explorations of the interface and the subsequent opportunities for creating new knowledge that reflects the dual persuasions'.

More recently, Durie (2012) has drawn attention to the United Nations Declaration on the Rights of Indigenous Peoples (UNDRIP), which advocates for the protection of indigenous knowledge.

The culmination of decades of work by indigenous groups around the world, this declaration was adopted by the UN General Assembly in September 2007, despite the opposition of four countries: the United States, Canada, Australia, and New Zealand. There is special emphasis in the declaration on self-determination for indigenous peoples, and there are articles devoted to indigenous peoples' rights to their traditional medicine and to maintain their own health and spiritual practices (Davis, 2010; UNDRIP, 2008). By 2010, the four dissenting countries had all adopted the declaration, which may open space for greater collaboration between indigenous healers and mental health professionals.

Partnerships between Indigenous Healers and Mental Health Professionals

Toby Minyintiri Baker speaks about the possibility of ngangkar̲i working alongside Western trained practitioners (Ngaanyatjarra Pitjantjatjara Yankunytjatjara Women's Council Aboriginal Corporation, 2013):

> As ngangkar̲i we really look at people's spiritual wellbeing—we look at how their spirit's going. If people are becoming dispirited or really exhausted, tired, unable to do things—we can recognise that in An̲angu[3] and work alongside doctors to help them.
>
> *(p. 192)*

Wiremu has used the expression tātaihono to refer to a close working relationship between an indigenous healer and a Pākehā psychiatrist. Here is a description of a similar working relationship from an Australian indigenous point of view. A ngangkar̲i, Wakupi Clem Toby, describes how his grandfather worked alongside a Western trained medical practitioner (Ngaanyatjarra Pitjantjatjara Yankunytjatjara Women's Council Aboriginal Corporation, 2013):

> My grandfather would watch Doctor Duguid working, using his style, but he was still very close to An̲angu, he was like their own kin. He was very knowledgeable. Our traditional ngangkar̲i doctors all went into his hospital to look around and they liked it very much. He had an open door policy and ngangkar̲i were welcome to come in and work alongside him. Often he would wait until the ngangkar̲i did their work before he looked at patients. He would give patients tablets and medicines afterwards. The ngangkar̲i were happy for him to work there and they were welcome to do their own work openly as well. It was open and the different doctors worked together.
>
> *(p. 240)*

Mario Incayawar, a Quichua medical practitioner and psychiatrist, co-developed a medical and healing centre in the town of Otavalo for his native Quichua communities in the Andean highlands of Ecuador (Incayawar et al., 2009). At this centre, Western-trained physicians work alongside yachactaita (Quichua healers) under the same roof. Patients have a choice about whom they see, and they tend to choose their practitioner based on their perception of their health problem. Physician practitioners sometimes refer patients on to their Quichua healer colleagues and vice versa. There has been joint research into llaqui, a Quichua name for a condition that has similarities to Western conceptions of depression and anxiety (Bouchard, 2009).

In the United States a Veterans Affairs mental health service at American Lake, Washington state, built a sweat lodge on their hospital grounds in the 1990s and employed a Native American spiritual advisor in order to add culturally specific aspects to their treatment programme for Native American veterans (Shore et al., 2009). Another centre in Colorado has developed formal and informal partnerships between psychiatrists and indigenous traditional healers for veterans living on remote rural reservations in nearby Northern Great Plains states (Shore et al., 2009). Clinical contact may be both in person and through videoconferencing. Shore et al. (2009) stress the importance of psychiatrists going out of their way to develop background knowledge of traditional beliefs and practices of the indigenous communities they are working with, actively seeking opportunities to work together, and becoming 'a serious student' of healing practices of the Native American culture they are working with. They emphasise the necessity of developing a trusting relationship with community members who are connected with the network of healers in indigenous communities. They outline several funding models that have been used to support Native American veterans receiving care from indigenous healers in their communities (Shore et al., 2009).

Although literature on psychiatrists and indigenous healers working together is sparse in the mental health field, a number of authors have suggested ways forward for partnerships between indigenous and nonindigenous colleagues in other settings.

Linda Tuhiwai Smith (2012) has written about the importance of addressing the legacy of colonialism in modern research partnerships between indigenous peoples and others, a process that she calls 'decolonization'. She describes decolonising as a long-term venture that involves each party recognising and peeling away successive cultural, linguistic, and psychological layers of colonial power in their work together. For such partnerships to work, there is a need for mutual respect and reciprocity, and 'a radical compassion that reaches out, that seeks collaboration' as well as an openness to new possibilities for a pathway forward (p. xii).

Leanne Simpson, a First Nations activist and scholar, points out that indigenous peoples in North America have been engaged in seeking justice, freedom, and political change for 500 years (Davis, 2010). She believes that there can be a role for partnerships with nonindigenous allies. However, in order for such alliances to be beneficial for indigenous communities, settler groups will have to 'decolonise' their connection with the environment by addressing unsustainable colonial practices in which resources are extracted from the land for short-term gain. They will need to decolonise their relationships with their indigenous neighbours by recognising indigenous sovereignty, not only over indigenous land and knowledge, but in many other domains, including indigenous authority over changes in the way these communities might interact. Transforming these patterns of relating could contribute to a future characterised by 'mutual recognition, justice and respect' (Simpson, 2008: p. 14).

There are many pitfalls, however, for Western-trained mental health professionals in embarking on such a journey, as there are many ways that indigenous viewpoints can be inadvertently silenced. Willie Ermine, a Cree scholar in Canada, has described an 'ethical space of engagement' based on appropriate ethical and human principles that may be formed when indigenous peoples and representatives of Western society are preparing to engage with one another (Ermine, 2007). Such engagement between indigenous and Western ways of thinking requires participants to be mindful of the extent to which Western therapeutic concepts tend to dominate indigenous paradigms and render them invisible. Simpson has advocated for indigenous peoples and their allies to reflect together on their collaborative relationships during times of relative peace, when there is time to 'retreat, re-evaluate, challenge and envision' (Davis, 2010).

One way to create such an ethical and reflective space is to attend to practices of cultural accountability. In recent years there has been increasing attention to these practices in indigenous and other services in Aotearoa (New Zealand) and elsewhere. In Chapter 1, I described my experience in seeing processes of cultural accountability in action at the Family Centre in the early 1990s. Based on the principle that 'the best judges of injustice are the groups that have been unjustly treated' (Waldegrave et al., 2003: p. 86), they developed collective accountability processes to address gender accountability (women's and men's groupings) and cultural accountability (Māori, Samoan, and Pākehā groupings). They identified that the process of addressing cultural concerns or injustices in the agency could be a very painful one, and that considerable vulnerability and trust were required in the relationships between the cultural groupings to find a way forward. The cultural accountability structure and process served these purposes and ultimately allowed for resolution of grievances, increased trust between the cultural groups, and creative solutions to the problems that the agency was attempting to address.

Allister

In writing my part of this chapter, I kept returning to this question: If we are talking about knowledge required for a health practitioner from a settler background to enter into a close working relationship with an indigenous healer, to what extent is it necessary to be mindful of the history between those cultures?

When I raise the history of colonisation between our peoples with Wiremu, he is happy to speak about his views on the impacts of colonisation; but I notice that he doesn't raise it with me. Perhaps he considers it discourteous. So I asked him if there was too much historical material in this chapter about the relationship between indigenous peoples and the peoples who have colonised their countries. His response was, 'No, leave it all in. People need to know about this'.

There is a danger for Pākehā or settler practitioners that coming to understand our own history in the eyes of indigenous peoples may render us paralysed, due to feelings of guilt or shame that we may experience. This is clearly a deeply unhelpful response. We need to step beyond this in order to be useful to our indigenous colleagues and their communities. In the words of Māori writer Patricia Grace (1992):

> Yet some Pakeha people, those with pride, are genuinely seeking. These few are coming to understand that what they can do in the interests of justice is to know themselves, to understand their own true history, which does not appear truthfully on pages of books, to understand the promises made on their behalf, to break their own silences, to search out the true meaning of racism and injustice, for which they are responsible only if they are inert. The seekers, the honest seekers, those taking measures, working out what can be done, are proud people who act from a base of self-worth, humility and dignity. They do not feel threatened but challenged. They know they need not feel ashamed or guilty, because they are claiming their own true heritage and their lives are honourable.
>
> *(p. 217)*

Wiremu

I think Patricia Grace's words resonate with what we are trying to do. She is saying that those with pride are seeking to understand what can be done in the interests of justice. For me, if I am seeking to be the best I can be for others, I first need to know who I am. Knowing who I am means understanding the history of my people. I need to understand what I am trying to achieve. And I then need to seek the tools and the means in order that I might be that. We need all of these different knowledge baskets. Together we are seeking to make sure that there is justice in this world. We choose to be on a path to seek the best health for those around us. We try our best to be the most hospitable to those who come upon us and to be the most respectful of those who remain around us.

Notes

1. Also known as Iroquois or 'Six Nations' people.
2. See Chapter 5 for a detailed example of a breach of tapu.
3. A<u>n</u>angu: Australian Aboriginal people who speak Western Desert Language.

References

Armitage, A. (1995) *Comparing the policy of aboriginal assimilation: Australia, Canada and New Zealand.* University of British Columbia Press, Vancouver.

Belich, J. (1996) *Making peoples: A history of the New Zealanders.* Penguin, Auckland.

Bouchard, L. (2009) 'The awakening of collaboration between Quichua healers and psychiatrists in the Andes'. Chapter 7 in Incayawar, M., Wintrob, R. & Bouchard, L. (eds), *Psychiatrists and traditional healers: Unwitting partners in global mental health,* pp. 79–91. John Wiley & Sons, Chichester.

Bringing them home: National inquiry into the separation of Aboriginal and Torres Strait Islander children from their families. (1997). Human Rights and Equal Opportunities Commission, Australian Federal Government.

Consedine, R. & Consedine, J. (2012) *Healing our history: The challenge of the Treaty of Waitangi.* Penguin, Auckland.

Crow Dog, L. & Erdoes, R. (1995) *Crow Dog: Four generations of Sioux medicine men.* HarperCollins, New York.

Davis, L. (ed.) (2010) *Alliances: Re/envisioning indigenous-non-indigenous relationships.* University of Toronto Press, Toronto.

DeJong, D. (1993) *Promises of the past: A history of Indian education.* Fulcrum Publishing, Colorado.

Deloria, V. (ed.) (1992) *American Indian policy in the 20th century.* University of Oklahoma Press, Norman.

———. (1999) *For this land: Writings on religion in America.* Routledge, New York.

———. (2003) *God is red* (3rd edn). Putnam, New York.

Duran, E. (2006) *Healing the soul wound: Counselling with American Indians and other native peoples.* Teachers College Press, New York.

Durie, M. (1998) *Whaiora: Māori health development* (2nd edn). Oxford University Press, Melbourne.

———. (2003) *Ngā Kāhui Pou: Launching Māori Futures.* Huia, Wellington.

———. (2004a) 'An indigenous model of health promotion'. 18th World Conference on Health Promotion and Health Education, Melbourne.

———. (2004b) 'Capturing value from science: Exploring the interface between science and indigenous knowledge'. Paper presented at the 5th APEC Research and Development Leaders Forum, Christchurch.

———. (2009) 'Maori knowledge and medical science: The interface between psychiatry and traditional healing in New Zealand'. Chapter 19 in Incayawar, M., Wintrob, R. & Bouchard, L. (eds), *Psychiatrists and traditional healers: Unwitting partners in global mental health,* pp. 237–49. John Wiley & Sons, Chichester.

———. (2011) 'Indigenizing mental health services: New Zealand experience'. *Transcultural Psychiatry* 48: 24–36.

———. (2012) 'Indigenous health: New Zealand experience'. *Medical Journal of Australia* 197 (1): 10–11.

Durie, M., Milroy, H. & Hunter, E. (2009) 'Mental health and the indigenous peoples of Australia and New Zealand'. Chapter 2 in Kirmayer, L. & Valaskakis, G. (eds), *Healing traditions: The mental health of aboriginal peoples in Canada,* pp. 36–55. University of British Columbia Press, Vancouver.

Dyall, L. (1997) 'Māori'. Chapter 3 in Ellis, P. & Collings, S. (eds), *Mental health in New Zealand from a public health perspective,* pp. 85–103. Ministry of Health, Wellington.

Engel, G. (1980) 'The clinical application of the biopsychosocial model'. *American Journal of Psychiatry* 137 (5): 535–44.

Ermine, W. (2007) 'The ethical space of engagement'. *Indigenous Law Journal* 6 (1): 193–203.

Field, M. (1984) *Mau: Samoa's struggle against New Zealand oppression.* Reed, Auckland.

Freire, P. (1985) *The politics of education.* Bergin & Garvey, Westport.

Grace, P. (1992) *Cousins.* Penguin Books, Auckland.

Haig-Brown, C. (2002) *Resistance and renewal: Surviving the Indian residential school.* Arsenal Pulp Press, Vancouver.

Hill, S. (2008) 'Travelling down the river of life together in peace and friendship, forever: Haudenosaunee Land Ethics and Treaty Agreements as the basis for restructuring the relationship with the British Crown'. Chapter 1 in Simpson, L. (ed.), *Lighting the Eighth Fire: The liberation, resurgence and protection of indigenous nations,* 23–45. ARP Books, Winnipeg.

Horton, R. (2006) 'Indigenous peoples: Time to act now for equity and health'. *Lancet* 367 (9524): 1705.

Incayawar, M., Wintrob, R. & Bouchard, L. (eds) (2009) *Psychiatrists and traditional healers: Unwitting partners in global mental health.* John Wiley & Sons, Chichester.

Johnson, T., Nagel, J. & Champagne, D. (eds) (1997) *American Indian activism: Alcatraz to the longest walk.* University of Illinois Press, Chicago.

Johnstone, K. & Read, J. (2000) 'Psychiatrists' recommendations for improving bicultural training and Maori mental health services: A New Zealand survey'. *Australian and New Zealand Journal of Psychiatry* 34: 135–45.

Kim, C. & Kwok, Y.S. (1998) 'Navajo use of native healers'. *Archives of Internal Medicine* 158 (20): 2245–49.

King, M. (1977) *Te Puea: A life.* Sceptre, Auckland.

———. (1983) *Whina: A biography of Whina Cooper.* Penguin, Auckland.

———. (2003) *The Penguin history of New Zealand.* Penguin, Auckland.

Kirmayer, L., Tait, C. & Simpson, C. (2009) 'The mental health of Aboriginal peoples in Canada: Transformations of identity and community'. Chapter 1 in Kirmayer, L. & Valaskakis, G. (eds), *Healing traditions: The mental health of Aboriginal peoples in Canada,* pp. 3–35. University of British Columbia Press, Vancouver.

Kleinman, A. (1980) *Patients and healers in the context of culture.* University of California Press, Berkeley.

Kopenawa, D. & Albert, B. (2013) *The falling sky: Words of a Yanomami Shaman.* Belknap Press, Harvard University Press, Cambridge, MA.

Kunitz, S.J. (1994) *Disease and social diversity: The European impact on the health of non-Europeans.* Oxford University Press, New York.

Lame Deer, A.F. & Erdoes, R. (1992) *Gift of power: The life and teachings of a Lakota medicine man.* Bear & Co, Santa Fe.

Lame Deer, J.F. & Erdoes, R. (1972) *Lame Deer: Seeker of visions.* Simon & Schuster, New York.

Langton, M. & Peterson, N. (1983) *Aborigines, land and land rights.* Australian Institute of Aboriginal Studies, Canberra.

MaGPIe Research Group. (2005) 'Mental disorders among Māori attending their general practitioner'. *Australian and New Zealand Journal of Psychiatry* 39 (5): 401–06.

Marbella, A.M., Harris, M.C., Diehr, S., Ignace, G. & Ignace, G. (1998) 'Use of Native American healers among Native American patients in an urban Native American health center'. *Archives of Family Medicine* 7 (2): 182–85.

McCarthy, C. (1993) 'Te Whare Marie bicultural unit Porirua hospital'. In *Tino Rangatiratanga and Māori Mental Health*, p. 5. Ministry of Health, Wellington.

McCreanor, T. (2012) 'Challenging and countering anti-Māori discourse: Practices for decolonisation'. Chapter 15 in Nairn, R., Pehi, P., Black, R. & Waitoki, W. (eds), *Ka Tū, Ka Oho: Visions of a bicultural partnership in psychology* pp. 289–310. NZ Psychological Society, Wellington.

Milloy, J.S. (1999) *A national crime*. University of Manitoba Press, Winnipeg.

Mohatt, G. & Eagle Elk, J. (2000) *The price of a gift: A Lakota healer's story*. University of Nebraska Press, Lincoln.

Moon, P. (2003) *Tohunga Hohepa Kereopa*. David Ling Publishing, Auckland.

Nairn, R. (2012) 'Psychology becoming bicultural—Māori keynote addresses: Was there something we missed?' Chapter 3 in Nairn, R., Pehi, P., Black, R. & Waitoki, W. (eds), *Ka Tū, Ka Oho: Visions of a bicultural partnership in psychology*, pp. 55–74. NZ Psychological Society, Wellington.

Newman, K. (2009) *Ratana: The prophet*. Penguin, Auckland.

Ngaanyatjarra Pitjantjatjara Yankunytjatjara Women's Council Aboriginal Corporation. (2013) *Traditional healers of Central Australia: Ngangkari*. Magabala Books, Broome.

Orange, C. (1992) *The Treaty of Waitangi*. Bridget Williams Books, Wellington.

Pere, R.T.R. (1984) 'Te oranga o te whānau: The health of the family'. Hui Whakaoranga: Māori Health Planning Workshop, Department of Health, Wellington. Cited in: Durie, M. (1994) *Whaiora: Māori health development* (2nd edn). Oxford University Press, Melbourne.

———. (1991) *Te Wheke: A celebration of infinite wisdom*. Ao Ako Global Learning New Zealand, Gisborne.

Pool, I. (1991) *Te Iwi Maori: A New Zealand population past, present and projected*. Auckland University Press, Auckland. Cited in: Consedine, R. & Consedine, J. (2012) *Healing our history: The challenge of the Treaty of Waitangi*. Penguin, Auckland.

Reynolds, H. (1996) *Frontier: Reports from the edge of White settlement*. Allen & Unwin, Sydney.

Reynolds, H. (1999) *Why weren't we told? A personal search for the truth about our history*. Penguin, Melbourne.

Robbins, J. & Dewar, J. (2011) 'Traditional indigenous approaches to healing and the modern welfare of traditional knowledge, spirituality and lands: A critical reflection on the practices and policies taken from the Canadian Indigenous example'. *International Indigenous Policy Journal* 2 (4): 1–17.

Royal, T.A.C. (ed.) (2003) *The woven universe: Selected writings of Rev. Māori Marsden*. The Estate of Rev. Māori Marsden, Ōtaki.

Scott, D. (1981) *Ask that mountain: The story of Parihaka*. Reed, Auckland.

Shore, J.H., Shore, J.H. & Manson, S.M. (2009) 'American Indian healers and psychiatrists: Building alliances'. Chapter 10 in Incayawar, M., Wintrob, R. & Bouchard, L. (eds), *Psychiatrists and traditional healers: Unwitting partners in global mental health*, pp. 123–34. John Wiley & Sons, Chichester.

Simpson, L. (ed.) (2008) *Lighting the Eighth Fire: The liberation, resurgence and protection of indigenous nations*. ARP Books, Winnipeg.

Smith, L.T. (2012) *Decolonizing methodologies: Research and indigenous peoples* (2nd edn). Otago University Press, Dunedin.

Somé, M. (1994) *Of water and the spirit*. Putnam, New York.

Statistics New Zealand. (2013) 2013 Census QuickStats about Māori. [Online] Accessed at www.stats.govt.nz/Census/2013-census/profile-and-summary-reports/quickstats-about-maori-english.aspx on 2nd December, 2014.

Stephens, C., Nettleton, C., Porter, J., Willis, R. & Clark, S. (2005) 'Indigenous peoples' health: Why are they behind everyone, everywhere?'. *Lancet* 366 (9479): 10–13.

Tamasese, K., Peteru, C., Waldegrave, C. & Bush, A. (2005) 'Ole Taeao Afua, the new morning: A qualitative investigation into Samoan perspectives on mental health and culturally appropriate services'. *Australian and New Zealand Journal of Psychiatry* 39: 300–09.

Tamasese, T.K. (2012) 'Interface of gender and culture'. Chapter 1 in Nairn, R., Pehi, P., Black, R. & Waitoki, W. (eds), *Ka Tū, Ka Oho: Visions of a bicultural partnership in psychology*, pp. 31–38. NZ Psychological Society, Wellington.

Tatz, C. (1999) 'Genocide in Australia', AIATSIS Research Discussion Paper No. 8, p. 10. [Online] Accessed at www.kooriweb.org/gst/genocide/tatz.html on November 10th 2014.

Tinker, G.E. (1993) *Missionary conquest: The gospel and Native American cultural genocide*. Fortress Press, Minneapolis.

Tui Atua Tupua Tamasese Ta'isi Efi. (2009) 'Tupualegase: The Eternal Riddle'. Chapter 18 in Suaalii-Sauni, T.M., Tuagalu, I., Kirifi-Alai, T.N. & Fuamatu, N. (eds), *Su'esu'e Manogi: In search of fragrance- Tui Atua Tupua Tamasese Ta'isi and the Samoan indigenous reference*, pp. 207–13. The Centre for Samoan Studies, Apia.

United Nations Declaration on the Rights of Indigenous Peoples. United Nations, March 2008.

Waldegrave, C. (2012) 'Challenges of culture to psychology—post-modern thinking'. Chapter 6 in Nairn, R., Pehi, P., Black, R. & Waitoki, W. (eds), *Ka Tū, Ka Oho: Visions of a bicultural partnership in psychology*, pp. 107–21. NZ Psychological Society, Wellington.

Waldegrave, C., Tamasese, K., Tuhaka, F. & Campbell, W. (2003) *Just Therapy- a journey: A collection of papers from the Just Therapy Team, New Zealand*. Dulwich Centre Publications, Adelaide.

Walker, R. (1990) *Ka Whawhai Tonu Matou—Struggle without end*. Penguin, Auckland.

Wieman, C. (2009) 'Six nations mental health services: A model of care for Aboriginal communities'. Chapter 18 in Kirmayer, L., Valaskakis, G. (eds), *Healing traditions: The mental health of Aboriginal peoples in Canada*, pp. 401–18. University of British Columbia Press, Vancouver.

3

HEY, MOKO, SLOW DOWN!

In this chapter we describe Wiremu's brief encounter with a young Māori woman who had left her whānau (family) behind and was living on the streets in our city. She was consumed with grief after the death of her beloved grandmother nine months before. Despite the brevity of Wiremu's intervention, this momentary conversation between them led to a dramatic transformation in Shannon's outlook, sense of well-being, and the direction her life then took.

Allister

Introduction to Shannon

From the first time I met Shannon, I very quickly formed the distinct impression that if she didn't approve of the direction that our conversation took, she would have no hesitation in dismissing me and leaving the room.

Shannon had been referred to our Māori Child, Adolescent and Family Service (Māori CAFS) by her care and protection social worker. She had recently turned 17 and was therefore legally of an age where the state would relinquish its care and protection duties; however, her social worker had some major concerns about her emotional well-being.

Shannon's world had been rocked six months earlier when her grandmother Makarita had died unexpectedly. Although her Nan had been ailing in the months leading up to her passing, nothing could have prepared Shannon for the shock of this loss. Makarita had been everything to her—she was like a mother, grandmother, and best friend all rolled into one. As is the case with many Māori tamariki (children), her Nan had been her primary caregiver throughout her childhood. As an infant she would sleep with her Nan in her bed, burying her face into her comforting embrace when she was in pain or distress. Later it was her Nan she would turn to for words of comfort and advice when trouble came looking for her in her early high-school years.

Shannon blamed herself for bringing raruraru (trouble) into her Nan's life in the last few years. Like a number of her 'mates', she had begun to reject adult direction. Her forthright and feisty style fuelled her rebellious responses, and she had begun skipping class. She joined her friends in smoking marijuana, and her absences became habitual. Despite her Nan's pleas, she was staying out all hours of the night with friends. By the time Shannon was 15, Makarita had grave fears for her safety out at night in the community. Aware of her own frailty, and convinced that she could no longer contain her granddaughter's behaviour, Makarita asked her daughter Cary, Shannon's mother, to step in and take over primary care.

Shannon was highly indignant about this change. Why should her mother have the right to tell her what to do, when it was her Nan she had grown up with? By the end of that year she had been asked to leave her college; however, the next year the whānau was unable to find another local college willing to enrol her. It was about a year later that her Nan's health took a sudden turn for the worse. Shannon knew that her Nan had been admitted to hospital. Just as she was making a plan with her mother to go and visit her Nan, they received a phone call from an auntie, in tears, telling them that Shannon's beloved Nan had just passed away.

When I asked Shannon about the tangi (bereavement ritual), she told me she couldn't remember much about it. All she could recall was a feeling of numbness. The shock of her Nan's death was compounded by the fact that she had not had the chance to say goodbye. In addition, she had become convinced that the trouble she had caused had directly contributed to her Nan's demise. And as time passed, the gnawing realisation that her Nan was gone became unbearable.

Just when it seemed things couldn't get any worse, they did. After repeated instances of Shannon running away from home, care and protection services removed her from her mother's care temporarily and placed her with a foster family. Shannon felt angry at the care and protection workers for robbing her of her family. She railed against the injustice of the situation, and her foster carers bore the brunt of her wrath. Before long several placements had broken down, and Shannon was feeling even more angry and despairing.

One night she secretly slipped out of her home. She had a rope and had been practising tying a noose. As she made her way down to the railway station, she thought about possible places where she might hang herself. Her world had literally fallen apart, and ending her life seemed the obvious way out of her despair. What stopped her in her tracks was a sudden vision of her younger brother Ben, aged 12, looking at her intently and commanding her: 'Stop!' It was at this moment that she realised that her brother and sister needed her and she couldn't go ahead with her plan to kill herself. A few weeks later, Shannon was referred to our service and she was seen that week for an urgent assessment by Tolly, a Māori nurse with our team.

In the three months leading up to her first contact with Māori CAFS, several of her whānau members had become concerned that Shannon was becoming depressed. She seemed sad all the time and would withdraw to her room when family members visited. Her familiar cheekiness had faded to the point that it was hard to even raise a smile out of her. She seemed to be sleeping erratically and, although she was previously known for her sharp temper, there was an edge to it that they now found alarming.

By the time of my first meeting with her, Shannon's family doctor had decided to prescribe an antidepressant medication for her. Shannon was in favour of this, as she wanted to feel better. In meeting with her, I agreed with her family doctor that she had easily enough symptoms of major depression to meet the criteria for this diagnosis. From that point of view, I supported the decision to offer her fluoxetine treatment. However, the losses that she had suffered over the previous nine months made it glaringly obvious that therapeutic avenues needed to be attended to if we were to be able to assist her further.

Shannon's nurse Tolly had an easy, self-effacing manner with adolescents and a knack for winning over even the most stroppy rangatahi (adolescent). Tolly was proposing to engage with Shannon using a Māori therapeutic approach known as Te Tuakiri o te Ora, which uses art and narrative methods to explore aspects of their personal and cultural identity (described in more detail in Chapter 7). One of the beauties of this method is that it can open space for a young person to explore painful territory without them feeling that they have to explicitly talk about it. Shannon seemed keen to engage with Tolly and she liked the sound of Te Tuakiri.

However, over subsequent weeks it was apparent that this plan was not going well. Shannon missed several sessions with Tolly and excused herself from home visits that had been arranged. Meanwhile she had decided against taking the antidepressant medication and threw it away. Before long, her latest placement with an aunty and uncle had ended because of some explosive rows, her erratic behaviour, and arriving home intoxicated. From here on it was hard to keep track of Shannon's whereabouts. We lost touch with her for several weeks, and her whānau had only patchy contact with her. On several occasions, however, she turned up after-hours to emergency services asking to see Tolly.

When Tolly finally located Shannon, she was living on the streets of Wellington. She had walked in to a local youth medical and social support centre, and they contacted us. They were aware of the group of young people Shannon was hanging out with and they knew the main area where these teenagers were residing, mostly sleeping rough. Shannon and her mates had had several run-ins with the police for stealing alcohol and food, and several times when Tolly caught up with her she was intoxicated.

When I was able to meet with her, it was clear to me that she was still very angry and, underneath her bravado and defiance, her pain at her loss was still very raw, compounded by the guilt she felt following her Nan's precipitate death. She hinted darkly that she might have suicidal thoughts, but didn't want to elaborate. By now, she was dismissive of the idea of counselling, as she had no hope that anything could make a difference for her. Shannon was convinced that her Nan was dead and gone and that nothing could be done to relieve the pain of her loss. She felt abandoned by her family and spoke angrily, using obscenities, about how little she cared about what she believed was their rejection of her (although, as we knew, her whānau was concerned for her well-being and had been at pains to get in touch with her). She made it clear that the only true friends she had were her companions during her days and nights on the inner-city streets. Sometimes she would turn up for breakfast at the 'soup kitchen' a few blocks from where they were hanging out. She said she was eating enough, but she spoke in a veiled way about fights with other young people in rival groups. Tolly offered to help her apply for a benefit and find accommodation, and she agreed, but later when Tolly returned to meet with her Shannon was not there.

In our multidisciplinary team we had several lengthy discussions about the pros and cons of using the Mental Health Act to compel Shannon to accept hospital treatment. What swayed us to delay this step was the way that she was prepared to engage with us and the rapport that Tolly seemed to be building with her. In addition, it was less apparent now that she had the same severity of depressive symptoms as when we had first met her, although it was quite possible that these were being masked by her bravado. Shannon was also demonstrating quite strong survival instincts and, despite her hints about suicide, there was no clear evidence that she was close to acting on any suicidal impulses. On the other hand we knew only too well there were many other hazards in the environment in which she was choosing to reside.

A number of worrying weeks passed when Tolly was unable to locate Shannon. We received reports from the police that she had been seen intoxicated with alcohol and solvents and that there had been frequent fights involving Shannon and her companions. Then one day, out of the blue, she turned up in an agitated state at our base at Te Whare Mārie in Porirua, some 20 kilometres away. Tolly was on leave, and another colleague, Lisa, who had also met with Shannon on several occasions, greeted her at the reception, where she was venting her frustration in no uncertain terms. Shannon's hair was unkempt and dyed a ginger and blonde colour. Her clothes were in a dishevelled state, and she seemed angry and distraught. Lisa responded calmly and skilfully managed to persuade Shannon to come with her to our whānau room, away from the waiting area. Lisa suspected that she was probably intoxicated, although it was unclear with what. However, Shannon was clearly not impressed that Tolly was not immediately available to see her. Because Shannon was in such an agitated state, Lisa knew that she would have to try to find out what had been happening with her, but when she asked about recent events, Shannon became angry again and before long was shouting at her.

Wiremu

I could hear Shannon when she arrived in the building. After some time I could hear her yelling at the clinician who was with her, and she was doing a lot of threatening and swearing. I was concerned that the clinician might need some assistance, so I made my way along the hallway to investigate. When I looked through the doorway, I could see a teenager that I hadn't met before. Her hair was wild and she was standing in the middle of the room facing Lisa, threatening and trying to intimidate her. She looked intoxicated. My first thought was about what I could do to defuse the situation.

However, as I came into the room I saw an old lady standing by the closed external door opposite me. Now I didn't know this old lady from a bar of soap. I could see her quite clearly, and she was leaning forward on a stick and she looked unwell. I could sense that she had some internal medical problem. As I looked at her, I became aware of her name, and I heard and felt a message from her for her mokopuna (grandchild). She was saying, 'Āta haere, e moko! Kia awhi au i a koe!' Shannon was still making quite a ruckus, but I said to her, 'Who's the Nanny standing here talking to you at the door?' She said, 'There's no effing Nanny there!' and I said, 'Well, her name is Makarita and she's saying: "Slow down, moko! I want to put my arms around you!"'

As I told her what the old lady had said, she looked stunned and went suddenly quiet. Her shoulders slumped and she was just staring at me with her mouth gaping open.

We now turn to Shannon for her account of what happened that morning.

Shannon Looks Back

I remember that day I first met Wiremu. Even though it was over four years ago, I can still recall it very clearly. I had turned up at Te Whare Mārie the night before and I had nowhere to sleep. At that time the external door to the reception area at Te Whare Mārie used to be an automatic opening door, so I slept in behind there. I was just coming down off some party pills I'd had the previous day and I wasn't feeling good. In the morning I headed off before the staff arrived. I just wanted to talk to someone. My mum was busy at work and at that time I wasn't allowed back at her house. I thought Tolly would be at Te Whare Mārie.

I remember I came back later that morning—by then the Whare was open, and I asked the lady at reception if Tolly was in. Well she wasn't there and then Lisa came out and asked me if I wanted a hot drink. I said, 'No, I just want to see Tolly.' But seeing as Tolly wasn't there, she said, 'Come with me and we'll have a hot drink and then we'll go to the whānau room.' And I was like 'Oh yeah', and we went into the whānau room and this felt alright to me and we were talking away. Soon after this Lisa said that she would have to ask me a few questions by way of assessment. Initially I was okay with this but then I got hōhā [annoyed] about some of the questions. Shortly after this she asked me a question that really riled me. I don't recall what the question was, but that's when I hit the roof! That's when I started going at her. At that time I tried to take off, but for some reason the external door in the whānau room wouldn't open for me.

That's when Wiremu came round the corner. As he walked in I heard him say, 'Kōtiro (girl), you need to slow down and breathe for a bit.' Then he went on: 'There's an old lady here and she's telling you to slow down, and to breathe'. I turned round and said, 'What fucking old lady, there's no old lady, there's only you and her.' At that time I was still angry about the question. I just wanted out. He goes, 'You need to breathe and to slow down and look at me.' For some reason I trusted him. So I looked at him. He goes, 'There's a beautiful old lady beside us here, and she's saying, "Please, just slow down!" At that time in my mind I was saying, 'I don't believe you. You're full of crap!' because I didn't believe that. But when he described what she was saying, it dawned on me, maybe it's my Nan. Every word he was saying to me, I was thinking, 'That sounds like her.' Wiremu even said something about her being unwell and having diabetes. It surprised me that he knew that.

There was no window, no door open, nothing. We were stuck in that room. But then I felt this breeze go across me. Wiremu said, 'Did you feel that?' And just then, I felt my Nan's hands go across my neck. She always used to do that, she used to touch my hair and my ears, and I used to hate it! And she did it in that room at that moment. That's when my attitude changed: I believed him. At that point I felt like my Nan was touching me. And he goes, 'She just wants you to breathe.' And I said 'Well, I can't, this is my Nan we are all talking about and I can't breathe without her.' And he said, 'Well, you'll just have to try.' He told me it didn't matter how much crap I got put through, he'd still be there for me. And I said, 'Sweet as' and he said, 'Just breathe for us.' And I sat there and told them everything, not what I thought they wanted to hear, but what I was really going through. And Wiremu, oh, he was the bomb! He sat there and took all of it in. All of the swearing, all of it. And I quite liked it.

My grandmother was a nice lady. But when her mokopuna (grandchildren) were in a bad mood, she could be in that mood too. She'd just sit there and tell us straight: 'Settle down.' Or she would go somewhere and buy something for us that we wanted. If we wanted some smokes or a feed, she'd get it. That's how she used to settle us down. We never used to talk to my Nan about problems, but if I was scared or in pain then I would always go to her. I was always the one in her bed. Even at 16, if I had nightmares and all that, I used to jump in and just snuggle up with her. I used to wake up in the morning and after she had taken off to work or wherever, I used to jump in her bed because I loved the smell of her. And next time I would wake up she would be at the bottom of my bed. She never used to go anywhere without telling me.

Later that morning, Wiremu asked me if I wanted some lunch. I was hungry so I said okay, and we resumed our personal talk in the kitchen. At that time I saw a lady putting corn in the microwave. I'd never seen anyone put corn in there like that. And I was going: 'What the flip?' and Wiremu was just laughing at me. Even though Wiremu had told me he had seen my Nan and that was how he knew so much about her, I was still trying to figure out if there was another explanation. I wondered if perhaps he knew my family and that was how he knew these things. So I asked him straight up: 'Do you know my family or what?' and he replied, 'No, I don't know your family.' 'Are you sure?' I told him all my last names, then I asked him, 'Do you know this person, do you know that person?' I told him where I was from. And he said 'No, I don't know them.' At the time I was thinking, 'Crap! This guy must be actually seeing someone, or he's playing around with me.'

I felt like he really was talking to my Nan. At one point I was crying because I wanted to talk to her, I wanted to hear what she had to say to me. I wanted to ask her advice: 'How do I get myself out of this shit place?' So I asked Wiremu could he say something to her for me and he said 'What's that?' and I said, 'Ask her to help me,' and he turned around and said, 'She says she will always be there for you, no matter what. "Keep your head up high and you'll do it."' That's one thing I missed was her advice. I always got good advice from her. I remember her yelling out to me when I was going on a school trip—I was captain of the netball team—and she said, 'Keep your head up high!' That day all I had been thinking was, 'We're going to lose, we're going to lose!' And she said, 'No, no, no. Stand on your own two feet. Let no one get in the way of what you want to do. Just do it! You've got a mind of your own. You just go and do what you want to do.' And when Wiremu was saying all those things about my Nan, the advice he was saying sounded just like her. That's when I realised I liked Wiremu.

A couple of weeks after that he asked if I would like to meet up with him for a coffee. I thought, of course I would! And when we met up we talked about everything. Even if it was just 'What did you do this morning?' We left nothing out. I always felt very welcome with Wiremu. The last time I saw him I told him, 'I feel privileged to have you', and he turned around and said, 'I feel privileged to know you, too!'

I didn't believe any of that spiritual stuff until I met Wiremu. I'm not the type of person to believe things I can't see. If someone said, 'There's a ghost there', I would say, 'Oh, whip dee doo!' I'm not the type of person to go to church. To my mind, you only live life once. So that means I don't believe in anything except myself and my family. But at that time, he changed a little bit of me. He made me feel like my Nan was there every day watching me.

About two weeks after that first meeting with Wiremu, I moved into a flat. After that I was slowly getting onto my feet. Later I had to spend a few months in prison, but even so, things had begun to change. My life was improving after that.

Allister

I wasn't present during Wiremu's meeting with Shannon; I learned about it sometime later. Frankly, nothing in my medical or psychiatric training prepared me for the notion that someone might be able to see and communicate with a deceased ancestor, let alone make use of such an extraordinary experience in a therapeutic way.

During the months when we as a team had been attempting to engage with Shannon, it had been clear to us that we might be able to help her if we could assist her to come to terms with her grief about the loss of her Nan. Conventional psychotherapeutic approaches for working through grief derived from the work of Elizabeth Kübler-Ross (1969) and others focus on working through a variety of emotional 'stages' that people may experience in response to their loss. But 'letting go' or 'saying goodbye' metaphors such as these can sometimes be experienced as aversive or unhelpful by people in grief. Another approach that I prefer is Michael White's work, 'Saying hullo again' (1988). This approach focuses on ways to assist people to reincorporate the lost other and that relationship into their life.[1]

In Shannon's case, despite our clarity about the source of her suffering, we had been wholly unsuccessful in assisting her with her grief. She had begun to trust her nurse Tolly, but there had been no way to engage her in therapy because of the tumultuous nature of her living situation, and she did not seem ready or open to a therapeutic endeavour. Yet it seemed that Wiremu's impromptu crisis intervention had a dramatic impact in a very short space of time. How can we explain this?

Shannon's description makes it clear that she warmed to Wiremu's personal manner and his way of interacting with her during the course of her first contact with him. Perhaps his status as an elder and his low-key and humorous style may have played a role in this. However, there is little doubt from her account that Wiremu's shocking observation that her grandmother was in the room with them played the greatest role in changing Shannon's experience of the loss of her beloved Nan. I am confident that in Shannon's case, even months of grief counselling would have been very unlikely to achieve such a change for her, even if she had been prepared to participate in it.

Perhaps Wiremu's approach to Shannon's predicament could be likened to a dramatic kind of reframe[2] in family therapy, or the compelling kind of new evidence that may lead to someone changing their way of thinking in cognitive therapy. But there is something unique in how Wiremu intervened here that I've never come across in any account of a Western type of therapy. At the outset Wiremu provided Shannon with evidence that her beloved Nan was present with them in the room. Equally vivid and mind changing, from her account, was the moment when she felt her hair being touched. Her description suggests that Wiremu was facilitating her experience at that instant when he said to her, 'Did you feel that?' Through this sequence of experiences, Shannon became open to the healing possibility that her Nan was still with her.

From a conventional psychiatric viewpoint, there is no scientific rationale to account for Wiremu's report of seeing Shannon's deceased Nan in the room with her. However, such experiences are commonly described in Māori and other indigenous traditional healing literature (Durie, 2009; Mark & Lyons, 2010; Moon, 2003; Parsons, 1985).

Wiremu

Seeing Shannon's Nan there in the room with us was not a surprise to me. I expect to see such things. I have this sense that perhaps Shannon's Nan was expecting me. The timing suggested to me that she knew I would turn up at that moment. She looked quite old to me, stooped by age, perhaps in her sixties. She seemed very concerned about her kōtiro and she had an expression of love. Part of having this matekite, seeing the dead, is the feeling that goes with the seeing or the hearing or other senses. In this case I could feel the love coming from her—there was a warmth. In other cases when there is some presence there that doesn't have good intentions, I often feel a chill; and in yet other situations I will see something and pick up a feeling of impending doom. But this time I definitely felt love coming from this Nanny for her kōtiro. The Nanny felt to me like a kaitiaki, a guardian who was watching over Shannon and trying to help her with her predicament.

Seeing her appearance, knowing her name, and knowing about her health came to me more or less instantaneously. All of these things were part of the message that I was given in order for Shannon to believe that her Nanny was there with her, not only present but wanting to help her granddaughter through her raruraru (trouble).

Te Hua (the Fruit)

In medicine these days a lot of people are talking about evidence-based practice.[3] I like to turn the idea of 'evidence-based practice' around and talk about practice-based evidence. I would ask what is the evidence that this intervention made a difference in this young person's life? And if there was a benefit, how was it helpful to Shannon? Did it help her with her mental well-being, her physical well-being, her relational well-being, and her spiritual well-being? And what evidence can you find in her life for such a change? It's what we call te hua, the fruit, the results of your labours. If she gets well in all these ways, then that's pretty good evidence, to my way of thinking, that the practice was effective for that person and their whānau. And I would say that in Shannon's case, the evidence we have is that she stopped living on the streets. She had to go to jail for a bit, but after that she changed her life around so that she was able to live much more harmoniously at home with her mother again. She stopped the drinking, sniffing, and drugging that she had been doing. She mended relationships. Now she has a supportive partner and is caring for two lovely tamariki in a way that she couldn't have done when she was in that state. To me, this evidence points to a transformation for Shannon. A renewal of her mind took place.

Still, I can't take any credit for this. It wasn't even me doing it. Whenever anything like this happens, it might have been somehow happening through me, but it can only come from my source. Without Io, without God, I'm nothing, and I couldn't do any of this.

The other thing is that the healing also comes from the young people themselves. All I can do is facilitate for people to go out and get the healing they need. We work in a collaborative way. What about the Nanny in this situation? She contributed to this outcome; in fact, it seemed like she was leading what happened. I don't go out of my way to look for tīpuna (ancestors) like this. Although I said that it seemed like she was waiting for someone, that was just my impression, and it might have been someone else she was waiting for. Perhaps there are others who would have seen her and passed on her message and this could have been as helpful for Shannon.

Kawemate (Bereavement Ceremony)

After that day when I first met Shannon, Tolly told me that the whānau were due to have a kawemate for Shannon's Nan. Often whānau will have an unveiling of the headstone about a year or so after the tangi. However, the kawemate is different. Kawe means to carry, and mate, in this context, refers to death. So kawemate is about carrying the grief of the whānau symbolically back to her tūrangawaewae, the place she came from. So let's say that Shannon's Nan was born in her local iwi (tribal) area, but moved to the city in her adult life. Perhaps she had lived in that city for 30 or more years, and the family decided she would be buried there because that had become her new home. What happens is that the family will get back in touch with people back home, those who couldn't make it to the tangi, back where she grew up, where she went to school, and a kawemate is arranged. At some point—months or it even could be a year or more after the tangi—the family will get together and gather a few photos and other mementoes that help with remembering the history of her life and connections in the city. Meanwhile, the people back home will be busy preparing for the visitors and getting ready to tell stories about those early years that they shared with her. This gives those who grew up with her an opportunity to grieve. The tangata whenua (people of the land) call the manuhiri (visitors) onto the marae, and they get together and tell stories about the person, just as they would at the tangi. And that's the process of kawemate. When this is complete, the formal grieving process has taken place.

And so when I heard they were planning the kawemate for Shannon's Nan, I knew that it would be very important for Shannon to be included to help her with her grief. But she had become so alienated from her family that I was concerned they might not include her. If she could be included, she would be with a lot of others crying and sharing their grief. Earlier she didn't have that chance, as she was in shock at losing her Nan and blaming herself, believing that she had somehow killed her Nan. So the kawemate is another opportunity to release all those feelings. I call this process of releasing and letting go whakawetewete.

Going back to the land that her Nan comes from is an important part of this. In te ao Māori (the Māori world), it is important to lay not only the physical body to rest, but also the spiritual. Her Nan's pito and whenua, which are her umbilical cord and placenta, were laid there when she was born. Spiritually as well as physically, Papatūānuku has been nourishing her during her life, and it follows that spiritually she must come back to where her pito and whenua were laid. It's a beautiful process.

Ka Rere Tonu Te Wairua (the Spirit Still Soars)

As we think back over Shannon's experiences, how can we understand what has happened here for her? Shannon knew her Nanny had died and, like many people, she was convinced her Nanny was dead and gone. It's like flicking the light switch off and you are suddenly in darkness. Naturally Shannon was in grief—her loss was very painful. Of course, grief can be deep enough to cause depression. A lot of people commit suicide because of grief. And often that arises from a certain way of thinking about death—that death is the end.

Well, my experience tells me that when we die, our spiritual part doesn't die. The physical body dies. We are formed from the earth and our body returns to the earth. But in regard to the spirit, death opens the door to another adventure.

I believe we are all first and foremost spiritual beings experiencing a human existence. So if the spirit is the foundation, then anything material is just added on to that. The body is the first thing added on. When you go and buy new clothes, you add that on. We add on cars and property and lots of other things. None of them are real! All those things will fade away in the end. If you took all the material stuff away, naked as a jaybird, you'd still have the same spirit. You might look at one another differently. You might say, 'Whoa! I didn't see that before!' And your body is just the same. This is something I just know and take for granted. Dying is a closure for this chapter. The body goes back to the ground, but the spirit lives on. And they say 'Ka rere tonu te wairua', the wairua still soars. It still flies.

So Shannon, who believes that her Nan is dead and gone, suddenly has a shocking experience that opens her to something new. She experiences something that changes her way of thinking about death. Before this, her Nanny had died, and she was stuck with her grief. Her only ways of coping were to get out on the street; to get 'out of it' on drugs and booze; to fight, steal, and get locked up. From one point of view you could say there was no closure for her—she couldn't move on from this loss. But from another angle, look at what gets opened up when her Nanny decided to return and reach out to her and say, 'Hey, tell my moko to slow down.' After this, Shannon begins to realise that her Nan is still very near; she hasn't left. Her Nan can now be very much in the picture. This knowledge opens up possibilities for her. She is then able to return to living her life.

Notes

1. Michael White's 'Saying hullo again' approach arose from his work with people who had been diagnosed elsewhere with 'pathological mourning'. While acknowledging elements that had been lost, such as the bodily presence of the person, he invited the grieving person to bring their departed loved one to mind with questions such as, 'If you were seeing yourself through the loving eyes of [your deceased family member] right now, what would you be noticing about yourself that you could appreciate?' Such questions were offered to assist the person to reincorporate their lost loved one into their lives.
2. A reframe is a method in which the therapist offers the client or family a new perspective, in the hope that seeing the problem in a different light might help them begin to overcome their problem.
3. Evidence-based practice refers to clinical practice in medicine, psychology, and other healthcare professions that emphasises the importance of basing clinical decisions on evidence from well-designed research studies such as randomised controlled trials.

References

Durie, M. (2009) 'Maori knowledge and medical science: The interface between psychiatry and traditional healing in New Zealand'. Chapter 19 in Incayawar, M., Wintrob, R. & Bouchard, L. (eds), *Psychiatrists and traditional healers: Unwitting partners in global mental health*, pp. 237–49. John Wiley & Sons, Chichester.

Kübler-Ross, E. (1969) *On death and dying*. Macmillan, New York.

Mark, G.T. & Lyons, A.C. (2010) 'Maori healers' views on wellbeing: The importance of mind, body, spirit, family and land'. *Social Science & Medicine* 70: 1756–64.

Moon, P. (2003) *Tohunga Hohepa Kereopa*. David Ling Publishing, Auckland.

Parsons, C.D.F. (1985) 'Notes on Maori sickness knowledge and healing practices'. Chapter 11 in Parsons, C.D.F. (ed.), *Healing practices in the South Pacific*, pp. 213–234. University of Hawai'i Press, Honolulu.

White, M. (1988) 'Saying hullo again: The incorporation of the lost relationship in the resolution of grief'. *Dulwich Centre Newsletter*, Spring.

4

GEORGE AND THE THING

In this chapter we show Wiremu's healing practice with a Māori teenager named George.[1] George was hearing a malevolent voice and experiencing seizure-like episodes that were disturbing his life. This chapter tells the story of how George's symptoms were resolved in a treatment process guided by Wiremu.

The narrative begins by introducing George and his whānau (family) and describing how they came to seek our agency's assistance. As the story unfolds, the reader is shown how these disturbing and extraordinary symptoms were culturally contextualised by Wiremu. Wiremu grounds these extrasensory experiences within a Māori body of knowledge, and George begins to feel reassured that his experiences are understandable and he will be able to take control over them. Within the recorded conversation of the single healing session, Wiremu provides cultural explanations for such afflictions, the factors that render young people vulnerable to them, and ways they and their whānau can protect and strengthen themselves.

In addition to giving Wiremu's cultural explanations for these afflictions, we show how George's symptoms are relieved in a single session.[2] The chapter concludes with a review of George's progress after the session and reflections of the participants.[3] George, his mother Arya, Allister, and Wiremu each provide commentaries about what took place and share their views on what was effective.

Allister

Introducing George

When I first met with George, aged 17, it was almost impossible to detect the cheeky sense of humour his mother Arya spoke of so fondly. The sparkle in his eye that she assured me was almost his birth right had been replaced by a tormented countenance.

I had already met Arya and her daughter, Makere, aged 15, who had been referred to our service four months before with depression and unusual seizure-like episodes. One month before that, George had begun having problems that were very disturbing for him and the family. At that stage the family doctor had referred him to our local early intervention for psychosis team, known as Early Intervention Service (EIS).

The problem appeared suddenly one night when George was out with friends. They had been drinking and were making their way on foot around a local inlet towards some nearby shops. Suddenly, to the astonishment of his friends, George jumped over the wall and plunged into the knee-high seawater. Within a few moments he was behaving so strangely that his friends felt compelled to call both an ambulance and his parents. Although George subsequently had no recollection of the incident, his friends initially thought he had injured his foot when he landed. However, he then began yelling, and when he calmed down, he spoke in an angry tone in a strange voice. His friends said he became unresponsive, jerking his arms wildly and erratically while remaining standing.

George's mother and other family members arrived at the emergency department shortly after the ambulance. He was examined soon after by medical staff, who carried out a range of tests. During this time, George acted in an uncharacteristically angry and agitated manner, at times yelling at the top of his voice. Lying on a hospital trolley, he tossed and turned restlessly. He was observed by his mother and emergency department staff entering into an unusual seizure-like episode inconsistent with epilepsy. He did not have a fever or other signs of physical illness, and the doctor's other examination findings and medical tests were normal—except for elevated blood sugar, which was consistent with his alcohol intake that night. His mother took him home soon after. Exhausted, George slept for much of the next three days.

A few days later he confided in his mother about hearing a voice that others couldn't hear: he first heard it the night of the hospital visit. He described it as a deep, masculine-sounding, female voice that seemed to be coming from outside his head. The voice sometimes told him to harm himself or others, and once told him to kill someone. It would comment on situations negatively; for example, after a minister came to bless the family home, the voice informed George: 'It won't work.' In addition, George became aware of a 'bad presence' next to him and intruding on him, which he associated with the voice. Hearing the voice sometimes occurred while he was having the seizure-like episodes. These episodes recurred over subsequent weeks, several times on some days and at other times with a day or more between them. During these episodes, he would become unresponsive and unable to speak and his muscles would tense up with jerking movements of his arms. George felt distressed by the voice and had trouble sleeping. He could not focus at school, and his family became progressively more worried about him.

When George was nine, he was diagnosed with diabetes, which shocked the whole family. He became habituated to the daily routines of skin-prick glucose tests and insulin injections, but recently he had become resentful of the restrictions and requirements. His friends always seemed to be able to eat when they pleased and stay up all night without any problems. It rankled with him that his life had become ruled by diabetes. His friends were going out together drinking, and he joined them. Some friends had taken up smoking marijuana, and in the months leading up to the onset of the problem, George had been doing so as well. Unsurprisingly, his attention to close control of his diabetes had slipped over previous months, and his mother had been concerned about his motivation for schoolwork.

The computed tomography (CT) head scan and electroencephalogram (EEG) brain wave recording organised by his psychiatrist at Early Intervention Service were normal. During an appointment, George had a seizure-like episode that lasted a few minutes. From a medical point of view, even though he didn't have other features of a major psychotic illness like schizophrenia, the voice that was so distressing for him seemed to be best explained as an auditory hallucination. Before the end of the interview his psychiatrist offered George a trial of an antipsychotic medication.[4] Willing to try anything to reduce or stop the voice, George accepted. At this point EIS referred him on to our Māori Child, Adolescent and Family Service (Māori CAFS), because they were unconvinced that George had a major psychotic illness despite the voice he was hearing.[5]

At our first meeting, I spent some time asking George and Arya about the difficult experiences they had been having. They left no doubt in my mind just how stressful a time this had been for George and the family. In spite of George's red hair and freckles, I knew that his whānau came from a very traditional Māori area. I wondered if they had been contemplating any cultural or spiritual explanations for his 'illness'. In order to explore this further, I asked them some questions to see if George had previous spiritual experiences in his life that might shed some light on his current predicament[6]:

Allister: In many Māori families, spiritual experiences are considered quite normal. George, have you ever had experiences like that?

George: (pauses, looks at Arya, then back at Allister) I'm not quite sure what you mean.

Allister: Well, for example, I wonder if you have ever had an experience of knowing something that you couldn't possibly have known through usual means, or perhaps a dream that ended up coming true in an uncanny way . . .

George: Hmm. Well. (looks at Arya)

Arya: Tell him about you and Makere.

George: You mean like the headaches and that?

Arya: (nods)

George: Well, I've always been pretty close to my sister. We often know things about each other. I can often pick up that she has a headache, or something else is wrong.

Allister: You mean you can tell by looking at her?

George: No. I have this feeling. Usually we are in different places but I can still tell. I get a headache for no reason, and at the end of the day I find out she got a headache too, at the same time. Sometimes I have wondered if it was a fluke, but it happens a lot.

Arya: What about that time with your dad? When he ended up in hospital way back when you and Makere were still at primary school.

George: Oh yeah. That time I was in class and I suddenly got a really bad pain in my hand. It was so sore, I was crying. My teacher told me to go over to the school office. I had only just got there when Makere turned up. She was all pale and holding her hand. The same hand. She said it was really sore.

Arya: I got this telephone call from the school office to say both my kids had turned up there and they were in pain. Shortly after that I got a call from the hospital and was told that my husband had been brought in by ambulance. He had badly injured his hand in a work accident with a skillsaw. I was pretty amazed when I figured out that the kids both got their pain in the same hand.

Allister: So how did you make sense of that?

Arya: Well, it's like you said before. I would see it as a spiritual thing. Other members of my family have those kinds of experiences. My mum knows about those things so I would discuss it with her. We both think that my children are aware in that way. George often knows if Makere has had a bad day or if she is unwell, or maybe he picks up that she is really sad about something. Then there was that time after Charlie died. Remember that, George?

George: Oh yeah. I'd forgotten that. (pause) Charlie was a boy who lived next door to us. After we had been to the funeral, we were all standing around while they were lowering the casket in the ground. Suddenly, I could see Charlie standing in front of me. I distinctly heard him say, 'Tell my family I am alright!' Then he was gone. It only lasted a few moments.

Allister: Have you had any other experiences like this over the years?

George: Well, sometimes I can feel my uncle around. My Uncle Hemi died last year and we were very close. But I can tell he's around me sometimes. It's hard to explain.

Allister: Can you say some more about how you can tell he's there?

George: Hmm. Well, it's a feeling. It's like I can feel him right here beside me, sometimes just behind my shoulder (indicates behind his right shoulder). He feels like a weightless weight. And he has a colour, a white and gold colour.

Allister: Is there anything else you'd say about that experience? Does it feel good or bad?

George: It's a good feeling. I know he is there supporting me.

However, George's recent experiences had a much more disturbing quality about them. In contrast to the benefaction of his experience of his uncle's presence, the voice was intrusive, hostile, and felt like a 'bad presence'. He located it just behind his right shoulder. He described it as 'dark pitch black on the inside and a dark shade of green on the outside' and 'like a 24-hour-a-day bully'. He was keen to rid himself of it. After two months on the low dose of his antipsychotic medication, the voice was reduced in intensity and frequency. The seizure-like episodes were less frequent, occurring about once a fortnight, but he still felt quite troubled by the 'bad presence'.

Experiences that George had recounted from his earlier years led me to suspect that he was a young person with a finely tuned spiritual awareness. His description of closeness to his sister, 'knowing' what she was feeling, the skillsaw incident, and his experience of 'seeing' Charlie at the burial reminded me of other Māori descriptions of spiritual experiences. In addition, his description of the voice as a 'presence' that he could locate in space made me wonder if there could be a Māori cultural or spiritual explanation. For this reason, I raised with George and his mother the possibility that we could consult with Wiremu. I explained Wiremu's role as our cultural therapist and expressed my trust in him and his work with other Māori whānau. George and his mother had no hesitation in accepting my suggestion and were keen to meet with Wiremu as soon as possible. When I spoke with Wiremu he asked to see them immediately.

Māori Healing Session

On the night of the consultation, Wiremu arrives off the plane from the Chatham Islands and sits down to a meal of kina (sea urchins) and fried chips in our staffroom. I meet George and Arya in our reception area, and Wiremu welcomes them in and invites the family to join him. The inviting aroma of the food seems to ease George's apprehension, and he eagerly accepts Wiremu's offer. After some light-hearted comments from Wiremu, George looks a little more relaxed.

I offer everyone a hot drink, then lead them into our meeting room. Once everyone is seated, I respectfully ask Wiremu to start our meeting with a karakia, and he responds by asking me to do it, which I do. We then have a round of introductions. As we do so, George looks very pale and I can see the tension mounting in his face and eyebrows. He introduces himself very briefly. His mother touches him reassuringly on the shoulder as she then speaks on their behalf.

When our introductions are complete, Wiremu comments on a tight, anxious feeling in his chest and a constriction around his throat. He wonders aloud if anyone can help him make sense of this. After a brief pause, Arya says that she knows that George is feeling worried about the meeting. George nods to confirm this but doesn't comment further. The smile that lit up his face briefly in the staffroom has now been replaced by the tormented expression I have seen at our previous meeting.

I ask the family if they would consent to us making an audiorecording of the session, and they readily agree.

Arya: Heck yes! If you can help someone else by what you learn, by your journey, oh yeah, we'll share that!

At this point Wiremu speaks about a number of concepts to clarify his worldview for everyone in the room:

Wiremu: Let me explain about 'wairua'. Wairua means 'two waters'. We are 65 percent water in our body. Most of our blood is made up of water. A lot of our brain is made up of water. So that's the inside part of us. But our outside part, which is our body, our 'tinana', the physical, is the outward expression of how we feel on the inside. So if I am thinking sadness, it is demonstrated by the tears. If I am thinking anger, it is demonstrated by my angry expression on the outside. If I'm anxious then you can see the physical manifestation of this in my outward appearance or behaviour.

Arya: Right.

Wiremu: So that's the wairua part; that's what we call the spiritual part of us. It took me ages to realise that.

Shortly after, Wiremu refers to the negative spiritual entity that he is now certain is impinging on George. Based on his intuitions about George, he has quickly reached the conclusion that he is a young person with spiritual awareness. Here he offers George and his whānau an explanation of why this negative entity might be affecting him at this time:

Wiremu: These things will try and hinder our journey. This is what I believe is happening now. Somewhere on your journey, George, you are going to come to the aid of others. This thing does not want you to help others. No matter when this takes place, even if it is years from now, you are going to lend someone a helping hand. So this thing will try to hinder your walk. Maybe you will help them just by talking to them. You might say, 'Oh, I remember this kooky fella, talking about this, talking about that . . .' (laughter) and suddenly they might go, 'Bing! Oh yeah, that's helped me.' It may be as small as that.

Wiremu explains that when a person's mauri (life force) and mana (spiritual authority) are weakened by negative events, family conflict, or drugs like cannabis, they become more vulnerable to negative spiritual influences. This is what Wiremu believes has happened to George. Now Wiremu outlines some key concepts to provide George with the knowledge and tools of his trade to take charge of this negative spiritual 'thing' that is affecting him.

Wiremu: Protecting yourself is about being selective about what you hear and see. You actually have the mana to do that. I just spoke about us experiencing the human journey, eh? We are spiritual beings first. There are a few more things I want to explain to help you to understand this.

Firstly, I talk about mauri. People talk about mauri as being a 'life force', and I talk about it as being in relationship with our creator, who is *the life force*. Next you need to understand about tapu. Tapu is the sacredness of that relationship. Finally we need to talk about mana. Mana is the authority given to you by virtue of that relationship with Io or God. This mana gives you the dominion over everything that walks, creeps, crawls, flies, swims, and anything that tries to hinder your walk. This means that you have that mana to actually kick this thing. Like I said, it's just that it knows you're 'not quite there yet', so it keeps going. You're saying 'Go on! Get out! Go on, p-off.' It might withdraw for a little while and then it will come back because it knows that you get really anxious about that kind of stuff. So, now, it's time for me to stop and let you ask a question.

(Pause. Silence.)

Arya: (to George) So what are you thinking? Are you thinking that this is making sense?

George: M-hmm.

During Wiremu's kōrero (explanation), George has been listening but has remained silent. Now there is a change in his demeanour. He has lowered his gaze. His breathing is becoming heavier. His shoulders and arms look tight and tense. Wiremu has noticed the change in George and asks him about it.

Wiremu: Are you getting anxious about it, George?

Arya: Come on, son . . .

At this moment all our attention is on George whose eyes are glazing over as he seems to be focusing on a distant point. His breathing is becoming very laboured.

Wiremu: Kei te pai. (It's okay.)

George is now having a seizure-like experience. He is breathing through clenched teeth. Both arms are very tense, and his right arm is jerking up and down in a taut rhythmical fashion, knocking against the table in front of him. Arya reaches across to grasp his left hand and talks him through the experience. The tone of her voice is strong and confident with little hint of the distress she must be feeling as she sees her son going through this yet again.

Arya: Do you want me to talk to you? Okay, darling, feel my hand. I am right here. Listen to my voice. Listen to my voice. That's right! I am right here, sitting right here beside you. Listen to my voice, that's right. You can do it if you have your eyes open and you can see me because I am right here—right here with you right now.

Rarely have I witnessed such an eloquent expression of a mother's care and protection for their child. I am spellbound by the calm and firm manner of Arya's speaking to George as she coaches him through this episode by encouraging him to listen to her and stay connected with the maternal power of her voice.

Arya: You can do it. That's right. Come on. Feel my hand. Squeeze my hand; come on; come on George! Can you hear my voice? That's right, good boy. There you go. Now open your eyes! We are all still here, alright? Awesome! You did it; you did it! Do you want a glass of water? A sip of water?

George remains seated but is leaning forward with his elbows on his thighs and now holding his forehead in both hands. His breathing is laboured. His whole body looks tense. Finally he lets out a long sigh. It is some moments before he manages to lower his hands and reaches out to take the cup of water that Arya is offering him.

Allister: It's a rotten thing, eh?
Wiremu: Too much, boy . . .

This episode has lasted only a few minutes; however, it feels so much longer. There is a pause in proceedings to allow George to recover from the episode he has just passed through. At last he breathes a little more easily. He now looks exhausted. When he appears to have recovered some of his equanimity, Wiremu speaks very softly and gently.

Wiremu: When we were sitting out there in the staff room, when you first came in, I noticed something about your eyes. I have this thing about looking at people's eyes because the eyes are the gateway to the soul.

I just looked at you briefly and what I saw looking back at me was actually not George. So this thing already knows that it's going to be *disturbed* . . .

As he speaks this word, Wiremu's tone changes markedly: from his quiet, clear, and focused manner of speaking, he now articulates this word in a deep, guttural tone.

Wiremu: So it will either try and make you say: 'Argghh, I am out of here, I am gone!' so that it doesn't have to leave, or it will make you react in a way that would, I suppose, upset people who don't understand what you are going through. And it's really lucky for you that she's here . . . (Wiremu points to Arya).

George: (nodding) Yeah!

Wiremu: . . . to kōrero, to bring you back to where you should be.

So this thing that I saw, when we were sitting out there, often we don't even have to talk for me to sense it. Actually, we all have that skill. It's just that some of us have developed it a bit better than others. So it's not something that I possess that you haven't got. It's just about you being able to learn about your mana, and when you do that, that thing will have to go!

But before we go tonight, I wouldn't mind having a karakia with you because it *definitely doesn't like that.* But we've already given it a bit of a shakeup. And it hasn't finished shaking yet. I have no respect for this thing, *this little gremlin!*

Arya: Yeah, I must admit George had an episode like that a couple of Saturdays ago and it was just me and George in the room. Normally I take a bit more of a calm approach like tonight, whereas on that Saturday, it pushed my buttons! So we were having a bit of a . . . (punching her right fist into the palm of her left hand). (laughter) Yeah? It wants to win? Yeah? My son? I don't think so!

Wiremu: Good job! That's the way to kōrero!

Arya: But I know what you mean about that moment when you looked into George's eyes. I have had that experience of looking in his eyes too. And I can tell when it's my son and when it's not.

Wiremu: You can see it, eh?

Arya: Yeah. I know when it is him looking back at me, and then it's like he's not there. It's not him!

Wiremu: Sometimes, when I use karakia, these things retreat. They try to hide. But I know it's there. I've already seen it. So yeah, you're onto it. You're onto it!

As I sense a pause in the conversation, I invite Wiremu to talk about his views on the effect of cannabis and alcohol on the mental and spiritual well-being of a young person who might have spiritual awareness. I have heard him talk about this many times, and I have a hunch that it will make more of an impact on George if he hears this from Wiremu than from another adult, such as myself.

Allister: Wiremu, one of the things you've said many times is that young people who have such a special gift are extra vulnerable to things like alcohol and dope . . .

Wiremu: Yep.

Allister: . . . and that could open the young person up to something dodgy. Do you want to comment on that?

Wiremu: It definitely does. What happens is that if you have got that gift, then drugs can open up a supernatural doorway. And just talking with you both, and just looking and feeling things, I know that you fellas do have that gift. So alcohol and drugs can open this supernatural doorway and then it can be really, really hard to close that doorway again so that we can be more selective about what we let in, or what we hear, or what we think, and what we see. It's like the tarutaru or drugs jam the doorway open. A lot of the time, I believe that's a possible reason for an illness like schizophrenia. There is a doorway that has been jammed open and everything just pours in. You know, without that, we can be selective about what we let in. There's a scripture . . . Have you been around church or anything like that? Because I don't want to be talking a foreign language . . . (Wiremu smiles)

Arya: (laughs)

Wiremu: . . . there is a biblical reference that talks about 'alienation in the mind' that pushes us away from what's reality, 'sometimes by evil works'. So that alienation thing could be from a traumatic brain injury or a chemical imbalance, or by evil works, which could be driven by an outside thing like taking drugs, self-induced stuff. You know, we can pour that in, and suddenly it's beyond our control. That's what happens to a lot of our people who are gifted. Like I said before, these things like to harass the heck out of people who they know could be using their gift to help somebody else somewhere down the line. They don't want that to happen. I know this because I went the same way with it. Until I learnt and matured enough to understand I needed to change what I was doing. Is that what you meant, Allister . . .?

Allister: Yeah . . .

Arya: I guess George wants to drink. And he was—up until he decided to jump in the inlet—he has done so a couple of times since because he has just found it too hard not to.

Allister: Because that's what all of your mates are doing, eh? Not drinking feels unfair, and the other thing is because George has diabetes he is already faced with stuff that he can't do sometimes . . .

Wiremu: Yeah, the old diet, and low sugar thing . . .

Allister: . . . it feels like life is not fair. I think it is totally understandable that you're wanting to do these things that your friends are doing. I guess what I'm keen for is for Wiremu to give you good information around your gift and how to look after it. And in a way it is unfair sometimes to have a gift.

George: But I guess that's sometimes how it goes.

Arya: Yes, it's a bit like that in life, when you get something good, you've got to give something up to get that goodness, eh?

Wiremu: Sometimes you don't want to either! (laughing) Sometimes, too, you're seen as being different. Like, I remember I would get cheeky and converse and still be around all my mates back then that were getting out of it and drunk. I would still grab a guitar or sing along with them and, of course, they wouldn't know the difference, whether I was drunk or not. But then at the end of the night, I would take them home, roll their smokes for them, and make sure that they didn't spill their beers. And later, when it got to the stage when I was actually using this gift to help people, I noticed they drifted away from me because suddenly I was seen as being different. Then I realised that you can't help who you are, you can't help what's been given to you, it's your thing in life. So, yeah, it is tempting. And the diabetes doesn't help either, eh, boy? It sucks, actually. But there is a reason for that as well.

But again, if you learn how to use your mana, that can help with an illness like diabetes too. I have done plenty of things that could have killed me. But I have this total thing, if you believe enough and if you can exercise this mana and say: 'I have authority over my illness, I have authority over it', 'Damn, you're not going to stop me doing what I want.' Last year I was in hospital for four days. I had a TIA [transient ischemic attack] which is like a small stroke, but by four days later I was much better and out of the hospital. For me this is about mana. I have my mana! (banging his fist on the table). Not that it matters with my wife! (laughter)

Arya: (laughs) That's a whole different thing!

Wiremu: That's a private mana!

Arya: (laughs)

At this point I am pondering possible ways that George can protect himself from a spiritual point of view. I am aware that he may not be conversant with many karakia in te reo Māori. However, Wiremu is often able to demystify such practices so that young people feel empowered to use them in their own ways.

Allister: Wiremu, I'm wondering if you could make a comment about karakia and how they might be helpful in this kind of situation. I know you would often use karakia to manage stuff like this, for protection. But it doesn't have to be in Māori, I'm guessing?

Wiremu: Nah.

Allister: But I'm thinking that whatever you do, it's got to feel right. I'm wondering if you have any thoughts about something George could do, just to protect himself or calm himself down over the next few weeks? Like a karakia or some other kind of thing.

Wiremu: The reason that I use karakia in Māori is that when you have a background in the culture, sometimes it can be very helpful. I remember this minister saying that he was asked to go to this house where they thought there was a wairua problem and he blessed this house and it got worse. These people rang him and said, 'Look, it's just gone really, really bad, worse than before.' So he went back and he took some others with him and they ghost-busted the house again. After this the people from that house rang him again and said 'Look, it's getting worse, it's worse than ever, things are breaking!' So he went back and he thought about it. This time when he blessed the house he did it in Māori and the thing left. The blinking thing couldn't understand English! It was an old—whatever you want to call it—a gremlin that had been around the family for ages; it couldn't understand English. He spoke to it in Māori and it disappeared. For me karakia is karakia. It's about people. It's about George's mana, you know, and so . . .

(At this moment Wiremu pauses, and the tone of his voice changes to a soft but very clear, low, and determined tone). See this thing I . . . yeah . . . (he laughs) . . . *This thing is gonna get it!*

Karakia is a universal thing, eh, and it's about protection and it's about telling the dirty stinking thing that you do have the mana to kick it around. Yeah. (pause). . . . Got a question?

George: No, I'm just listening . . . listening, especially when it's good stuff to take in.

Wiremu: Too much, boy, too much.

George: This stuff gets pretty tiring.

Wiremu: Yeah, of course it does, course it does. I can imagine that it does.

Arya: The big thing is, whether it lasts 30 seconds or three hours, he's zonked afterwards.

Wiremu: Oh, it's tiring alright. I mean just in those few seconds at the beginning when I felt this anxiety in my chest and throat, when I felt the anxiety attack, oh, it wasn't nice, and I only experienced it for a short moment. That's why I asked about it, when I felt tense around here (indicating his chest) . . . you know.

George: I have been pretty tired in the last weeks. Like, I've got home from school, and I've just gone to sleep. Like I'm really trying to keep this thing out. I'm trying to hold this thing off . . .

Arya: So just being yourself is getting . . .
George: . . . pretty tiring . . .
Arya: . . . really tiring!

At this moment I recall a conversation from my first meeting with George, and I ask Wiremu to comment on it.

Allister: Something else you mentioned, George, is that you had an uncle who died a while ago, eh?
George: Yeah.
Allister: . . . and you can still feel him around sometimes? Is that still happening at the moment as well—in the last couple of weeks?
George: Yeah.
Wiremu: How long ago did he die?
Arya: About July last year.
Wiremu: What sort of relationship did you have with your uncle?
George: A great relationship. Me and my uncle were very close.
Allister: I'm guessing that he is keeping an eye on you?
Wiremu: Yeah, I was just going to say that.
Allister: Is that a good thing to have?
Wiremu: Yeah. We all have our kaitiaki, our guardians. We all have them around. This is why it's important for us to understand about our whakapapa, our genealogy.

By now Wiremu is coming to the conclusion that this current problem has been brought about through some unresolved intergenerational issue that has negatively affected George and the family in addition to his cannabis use.

Wiremu: It's often our ancestors who try and protect us. There is a lot that I could explain about this. A problem could come about if there were things I needed to let go of. If people had hurt me, and I was angry, and I was bitter, and I was starting to get ill because of it—which you can get—then I would need to release them.
George: What?
Wiremu: I would need to release them.
Arya: I was just thinking. (She turns to George) This comes back to the kōrero we had about the family bust-up, at Christmas up north. You and your sister both came back from that family gathering 'broken', and that never got resolved. Maybe George's problem may have manifested in this way. We've all sat down and gone 'Why both the kids?' Why both my kids? I have only got two, and both of them have had this downward spiral. Makere even has these similar episodes. Hers are a bit different, but they both started having them within a month or so of each other.

Now Wiremu introduces a healing ritual that he uses with many whānau to address unresolved intergenerational conflict, even when it may involve generations who have passed on many years before.

Wiremu: I call that process whakawetewete, which is to give away, to release, to give up. Now, just going back to your whakapapa, if we manage to do that whakawetewete, then what happens is it's no longer our burden to carry, but the burden of our whakapapa, our ancestors, to step in there and say, 'Move over, we'll take over from here.' That's the thing, and it works, it really does.

See, there is another kōrero too, a biblical reference. I use that because I don't understand English very good, so I use those references. It talks about the sins of the forefathers visiting upon the sons, or upon the children. If something has not been resolved in the generation before or the generation before that, or even further back, if there has been no reconciliation, or restoration, or reparation, then that could turn into a curse upon the family. And it will visit upon the generations, until it's (gesture of chopping onto the middle of his hand) cut off. So that's what happens.

Arya: Yep, we can't just quite figure out which side of the family this has come from and exactly what we need to do . . . It's all making sense though. Me and my mum talked about that. See we talked about the fact that if there is take [cause], if there is raruraru [conflict], it will find an outlet, and it's my damn children, and it's not fair! But we don't know . . .

Wiremu: You can't pinpoint it . . .

Arya: We can't pinpoint it so we are not sure how to proceed.

Wiremu: You know when I talked about hurts—the fact that your children have suffered something that you can't understand, that's got to be hurtful. So in trying to resolve this thing, look at all the stuff that's hurt you, including the fact that the kids got whacked by something you don't understand. Anything that has hurt you at any time, write it down. Also write down all the times that you might have hurt others. Once you've all done that, then you can go down to the beach together and have a ceremony where you take these bits of paper with all these hurts on and make a fire and burn them. And that way you can release it. You can say, 'I just give this up, to the universe, to whoever, to take care of this burden. It shouldn't be mine alone.' Eh? In doing that you are giving your burden back to your whakapapa [genealogy/ancestors].

Same with you, boy. You know this thing that's happening to you? You need to let it go. Just say, 'I release this, I forgive it', because it doesn't understand and you certainly don't know where it's coming from. And just say, 'I give that up, it's not my burden . . . it's not going to be my burden anymore.' Your tīpuna [ancestors] will take care of you after that. Because it is about your mana.

But before we close up, would you give me permission to karakia for you?

George: Yes.

Wiremu: Too much, man, thank you very much. Is there anything else you wanted to ask?

George: No, it's good.

Wiremu: You can always refer back to Allister if you need to know a little bit more. But all that is required is writing down the hurts, the situations, the times. You know, people have done things that really hurt me. I remember I had to let it go. And I think I hurt a lot of people, too, and I had to let that go as well. So you have the opportunity to cut that (gesture of cutting) thing of where the sins of the forefathers visit upon the children. We talk about utu, eh? In the Bible they talk about utu, 'an eye for an eye, a tooth for a tooth'. We are almost the same. Utu means we get paid back for what we do. They used to have a process called 'muru'. If you pinched my cow, rather than kill you, I would say, okay, every first-born calf you have every year, I would get it until I think you have paid me back. And that was quite good justice, to go and do that. If that never happened—if, like I said, there was no reconciliation, reparation, or restoration—utu went to mākutu, which was the curse. Yeah, that's what happened.

Now I made that up! Nah I didn't. (laughter)

Arya: It sounded good! (laughter all round)

Wiremu: Okay. I'm just going to come around and karakia for you.

Wiremu stands up and walks around behind George and lays his large hands on George's shoulders and head. George takes a slow breath and it looks like his shoulders have relaxed during all this conversation. He looks pleased that Wiremu is going to karakia for him. As Wiremu begins the karakia, he is standing behind George. He pauses for a moment, then speaks softly:

Wiremu: (Karakia) E Pā, Te Matua, I just pray right now, for your aroha, for your strength, for your courage, and Lord I just pray for your protection. I ask in your name that anything that is not of you, in this young man's life, in this young man's mind, that it shall come off. I speak not in my own authority, but the authority of the Creator, of my source . . . that anything that is not of you, shall leave. Give him rest, give him rest!

Lord, I just pray for this whole family, I pray that you protect and guide them.

Come off, come off, come off, come off.

Thank you, God, I don't have to say any more, you take care of it, by your holy spirit. Tonoa mai tō wairua tapu, tukuna mai, thank you Lord, thank you . . . Korōria ki tō ingoa tapu. Āmine.
(pause)

Just lean back a bit George . . . (Wiremu repositions his hands on George's shoulders) There is another biblical thing that always talks about the renewing of the mind. I just pray that you impart that power that has been given. The karakia where you lay hands on those who are afflicted, that they might be set free. I just pray for that right now, right now for the renewing of the mind. Thank you Lord, thank you Lord.

Wiremu holds his hands there for a long moment. Then he walks back around to the other side of the table and sits down again.

During the karakia I notice that the hairs on the back of my neck feel like they are standing on end. I'm still aware of this tingling sensation as Wiremu sits down. There is silence as everyone allows this moment to sink in. Arya is looking at George, searching his face for a sign of how this experience has been for him. George looks pale and exhausted, but there is a slight smile on his face and an expression of relief.

Wiremu asks me to give him an update on how things are going for George as soon as I see him the next time. I suggest to George that he continue his risperidone medication unchanged until we meet in a few weeks' time, and he readily agrees to this. We confirm our next appointment time. As we all stand and walk out, George is joking with Arya and there is a lightness about his demeanour that I haven't seen before. As they leave the building, they are chatting about a plan that George is hatching for the weekend.

George's Progress after the Session

After two postponements from the family, the next follow-up appointment was two months later. As it happened, Wiremu was available to catch up with the family at that time as well. It was a pleasure to see George and he was in good spirits—clearly his sense of humour had returned in full measure. George relayed that he had stopped his antipsychotic medication soon after the first session with Wiremu. He did this because he had gained over five kilograms of weight on this treatment, and this weight gain had been interfering with his blood sugar control. He had also accepted Wiremu's view that his psychotic-like experiences had a spiritual origin.

He described to us one moment when he had been aware of the bad presence around but had not heard the voice and had been much less bothered by it on that occasion. He hadn't heard any more voices or experienced any further seizure-like episodes. He said he had felt 'uplifted' after meeting with Wiremu. He was feeling much more positive and confident in himself. He had been reluctantly avoiding drugs and alcohol and was gradually accepting that this was necessary for his spiritual well-being and his diabetes control, despite his friends' drinking habits.

Four and a half years after the session with Wiremu, Arya contacted me after George had a further seizure-like episode at work. She asked if it was possible for them to see Wiremu again. I arranged for Wiremu to ring the family. He spoke with Arya and George and, after hearing their description of the recent experience, he reiterated his advice from the original session and offered to karakia for George. Over the next six months, up to the time of this book going to print, George was working and did not require further mental health assistance.

We turn first to George and Arya for their reflections on the experience of meeting Wiremu and how they perceived his approach to what had been a very distressing problem for George and the whānau.

George

The five months prior to meeting Wiremu was a very freaky time in my life. It felt like a bad nightmare. I was feeling terrible all the time. I was always having to think about the thing in my head. I was not in a good place with myself. One of the scariest things was that before we met Wiremu, no one really seemed to know for sure what was going on. The professional people we met were kind and they all had ideas, e.g., it could be psychosis or it could be something else, but I was sitting here with it for months on end and I still didn't know what it was.

One of the things that really helped me about Wiremu was that I understood what he said. It was curious because when he talked about the problem, his ideas felt right to me. He gave me a spiritual explanation, and there was something in me that knew that he was right even before I understood intellectually. I was like 'Yep! I'll go with that.' And then he would explain it more and I was like: 'Now I know, and I feel what he is saying is good.' It was like putting it out there, talking about it, putting it in its place, giving it substance. And as Wiremu said, giving the 'it' substance helped me to kick it in the ass!

In the two months since seeing Wiremu, the weight has lifted off me and I feel a lot better in myself. I feel like I'm on my way to becoming stronger. Now I am able to keep myself well.

When I first walked into the room with Wiremu, it felt like whatever was in me just sprang out. It was like it was being fought with. It felt to me like there was someone else in the room with enough mana to share this with me.

When Wiremu did the karakia with me, I felt it diminish. It was like this thing went from being completely there to fading. I just felt better physically and spiritually. And now I can feel real good in myself in all ways!

Interestingly, there was one time when I was aware of the voice again, about four weeks after seeing Wiremu. It felt as if someone I knew walked past quite quickly and I kind of glanced at them and thought, 'Oh, I know that guy,' and then they were gone. I kind of noticed it and thought, 'Oh there's that voice.' But I felt it more than heard it.

One thing I have really learned is that *I can just let things go.* Recently I went from having a girlfriend to not having one. She texted me and said, 'Oh we could try this again later', and I could have been very down in the dumps about it, but after being through all this and Wiremu's kōrero about releasing things, I was like, 'Oh well, that's how it goes, I just have to let it be.'

Arya

George was uplifted after seeing Wiremu. Beforehand, even though he was very good at communicating what was going on to me, you could see the burden. You could see that the things that were going on were weighing him down, and perhaps the lack of knowledge or the feeling of powerlessness weighed on him. But during the meeting with Wiremu and Allister, I could see a change in George's body language. His posture picked up. With Wiremu there, it seemed to me that he had the mana to share this spiritual burden that George had been carrying. I felt like we didn't have to do this on our own anymore. It was like, 'Ahhh, what a relief!'

George is a really funny guy. His natural personality is to be cheeky, to be smart, to see the funny side, to make little comments that will always make everyone else laugh. And that had gone. It was that type of stuff that returned after that session. He was soon back to his old bright, bubbly personality.

For me the biggest thing about meeting with Wiremu and talking with him was seeing that it all felt right and made sense to George. It felt right and made sense to me, but watching George, I could see that it felt right and made sense to him, too. And with that package then I thought: 'Hah, yeah, we've got it, we're onto it!'

I didn't mind what was wrong with my son. If it was psychosis and he needed medication, fine, so be it. But if it was wairua and he needed to tap into that and set his spirit right, and maybe acknowledge his tikanga (Māori customs), then that was okay too. So for me I didn't mind which avenue, which road we had to go down. We needed to go down the one that had well-being at the end of it for my son. It became clear during our session with Wiremu that this was a bit of a battle of his wairua. It was a spiritual thing that he needed to work through. After that night it fell into place. It's now two months since our meeting with Wiremu, and although I know George is not 100 percent, he's well on his way to it.

When Wiremu did the karakia that was interesting for me. I'm not a particularly religious person. I don't go to church, but I must have done enough Sunday school to know what Wiremu was talking about. I liked what Wiremu was praying about. He was asking for a 'new mind' for George. This made heaps of sense to me. If you are going to pray for something, yeah, let's pray for a new mind! So it was logical.

Although I'm not sure about the religious part, for me the spiritual side of prayer is purifying. It has a cleansing effect. There is a reason why you pray before you eat. Especially for me, being Māori, all the different protocols and processes we follow are about tikanga. And respecting tikanga doesn't necessarily mean to be religious. They don't actually go hand in hand like they do in a lot of other cultures. You might meet a Māori on the street and they don't believe in God but they will still pray or they will still observe the tapu rules on a marae. All that kind of stuff is important because it's cultural. It's what you do.

Recently I've been very interested to see how well George has coped with the end of his relationship. I spoke with him about what Wiremu predicted for his future. I told him, 'This is another learning curve; this is another tool to put in your kete, for whenever time calls upon you to help another.' Wiremu said he's going to be there to help someone someday. All the experiences he has between now and then will help him when the time is right for that.

George: Five Years after the Session with Wiremu

I'm 22 now and for the last year I've been working (at a fast-food outlet). Mostly I'm good, but about six months ago, I had a few of those episodes. A couple of times, my boss noticed and he moved me out of the work area and gave me space to calm down. I told him it was my diabetes, but it wasn't. The third time it got much stronger. Luckily he called my mum. Where we work is very cramped, and there are about a dozen people working close to me and lots of customers coming in and out. And I'm sure there was someone there who was bringing something in with them to work, something spiritual. Normally I can resist those things—I use my awareness to stay calm and take care of myself. But that time, I was starting to get stressed, and so I ended up blocking everything out. I switched myself off to it, and my guard was down. So I think that's how it got to me. And I had one of those seizure things. But since then it's been okay. I've been back to normal.

The thing that was with me when I saw Wiremu hasn't been around for a long time. Maybe I felt it around briefly about a year ago, but not since. I don't hear things. Mind you, I make a point of not listening in. But I still feel heaps of stuff. Just the other day I went from having a normal day, feeling real good, to suddenly feeling really upset. I had tears in my eyes and I didn't know why. So I texted my sister: 'You're not alright, are ya?' She responds: 'Nah!' It turns out she was having a feud with her boyfriend at their new house. She told me: 'I just want to come home!' My response was: 'Yeah I know, I can feel it!'

As for seeing things, it's not quite like that. It's not exactly visual seeing. I call it, 'see-feeling'. Like seeing without using your eyes. I can do it with objects. The other night we were outside the netball club in the carpark. I was standing by the car waiting for Mum to finish her cigarette, and it was pitch black. I could feel something there on the ground behind me. I turned around and peered onto the ground and reached down for it. It was a taonga, a greenstone pendant. And normally, we always know that if you find something like that, you leave it where it is. Don't pick it up. But this time, it felt like 'closeness'. And I knew that it was the right thing to take it home. So I did. And I texted my sister and my cousin about it, and sure enough my cousin had dropped her taonga there the night before. But she hadn't told anyone and didn't know where she'd left it.

Arya: Five Years after the Session with Wiremu

George and I have talked a lot about his spiritual awareness over the last five years. It's almost like something else that he has had to learn to manage, like his diabetes. And he seems to find talking about it helps him become more aware of when it is affecting him and how to best manage it. I notice these days that he generally doesn't allow himself to be caught off guard. He uses his awareness to protect himself. He can walk into a room and might think, 'Yep, I don't like what you've got happening—I'm off!' and he'll remove himself from being around that person or place. I try to make sure our household is peaceful. If we had a world war three household, it would drive him nuts. Because he's tuned in, he would be affected by all that raruraru, even if there weren't noisy arguments going on.

I haven't forgotten what Wiremu said, that if George wanted to, he could choose to close himself off from the wairua stuff. So once every six months I ask him if he'd like to go down that path. But he always declines. He maintains that life would be too boring.

Allister

As George's psychiatrist, part of my job was to advise George and his family as to whether his experience of the voice might indicate that he was suffering from a serious psychotic illness. The voice did seem consistent with an auditory hallucination, which by definition implies that he was hearing something for which there is no basis in reality. Interestingly, in psychiatry, we don't have language to describe an experience that is unseen but may be perceived by more than one person. In this case, both George and Wiremu could perceive the same entity impinging on him. Is this enough for us to say that it isn't a hallucination but represents some kind of entity that is based in reality? If not, who else would need to be able to perceive it for its veracity to be confirmed? If it is enough, what kind of language can we use to describe this kind of perceptual experience?

Many Māori and Pacific young people I meet in my work describe extraordinary perceptual experiences at some time in their lives when they haven't been using substances. Frequently these experiences aren't distressing for them, and they don't wish to have any help to modify them. If Wiremu and other Māori colleagues are right and some of these young people have a degree of spiritual awareness beyond the usual, then it follows that we as clinicians may be able to ask them questions that will help us and them to identify this pattern in their lives. Earlier in this chapter there was an example of dialogue that illustrates such a line of questioning. Further examples are offered in Chapter 8. In addition to George's unexplained distressing symptoms, his and his mother's responses to these sorts of questions convinced me to ask the family if they would like to consult with Wiremu.

However, returning to the subject of how George's symptoms and experiences can be categorised diagnostically, his experience of the voice seemed to reduce in frequency and intensity after he had taken risperidone for several weeks. He had also begun to smoke cannabis over the previous six months, which is a common trigger for a first episode of a psychotic illness (Arseneault et al., 2002). At the same time he didn't have other symptoms indicating a psychotic illness.[7]

I was even more puzzled by George and his mother's description of the seizure-like episodes. These episodes seemed to be consistent with a type of nonepileptic fit known as pseudoseizures. He was not collapsing to the ground, and although he was having some jerking rhythmical movements of his limbs during these episodes, he was not fully unconscious and other features that would suggest an epileptic cause were not present. I witnessed one of these episodes in my first meeting with George and his mother, and despite George appearing unresponsive for a few minutes and the jerking movement of his arms, which was more in one arm than the other, he remained more or less upright in his seated position on the couch. He appeared to be listening to his mother's voice as she talked him through it. However, it was clearly a very unpleasant and exhausting experience for him.

From a psychiatric point of view, pseudoseizures are commonly viewed as a kind of dissociative symptom in which the affected person may be experiencing some kind of serious psychological conflict that they are unable to resolve or even put into words (Bodde et al., 2009). The mind's way of coping with this is to express the conflict unconsciously with disturbed behaviour in a form that resembles a seizure. Often children with pseudoseizures may have a family member or someone known to them suffering from epileptic seizures (Sadock & Sadock, 2005). In addition, pseudoseizures and other dissociative symptoms often occur when a young person has experienced major trauma in their life, such as war, or sexual or physical abuse. In George's situation, he did not report any of these kinds of traumatic experiences. Nor did he show signs of the kind of internal conflict that would provide a coherent psychological explanation to account for dissociative symptoms. There was no one with epilepsy or psychosis in George's family, and the only person with any similar seizure-like episodes was his sister, who had her first episode one month after his.

From a traditional psychiatric perspective it could be argued that Wiremu's spiritual explanation for George's symptoms is implausible. Although the voice that was tormenting George and the pseudoseizures both ceased after his first meeting with Wiremu, alternative explanations for his improvement might include his avoiding cannabis, the effect of the antipsychotic medication (even though he stopped taking it), or even the power of suggestion in Wiremu's work with George. However, although brief psychotic disorders that clear up spontaneously are well described, true psychotic symptoms such as auditory hallucinations of this intensity that have persisted for over five months might not be expected to suddenly remit when antipsychotic treatment is stopped. They aren't usually considered to be susceptible to the power of suggestion, either (Sadock & Sadock, 2005). Alternatively, a psychodynamic psychiatry perspective could take the view that George's vivid experiences may have resulted from some intrapsychic conflict. The resolution of his symptoms from that point of view could come about through some element of his encounter with Wiremu that assists him in finding resolution to this conflict (Gabbard, 2005).

What was compelling for me about Wiremu's assessment and treatment of George's situation was Wiremu's clarity about what he perceived was going on for George, his confidence that his intervention could help, and the positive results that transpired. Most compelling was George's description of the change that he experienced. George's account of the nuances of the 'thing' tormenting him included its location in space next to him, its colour, and the malevolent intention that was congruent with the content of the voice he kept hearing. Risperidone treatment had dulled the intensity of the voice, according to George, but had not affected the other aspects, whereas Wiremu's intervention seemed to banish the voice entirely. Moreover, for the first time George and his mother said that they'd heard an explanation that made sense to them. They felt much more hopeful and empowered to take action against the 'thing'. Wiremu had concluded that there was an intergenerational problem in the whānau that would account for the problem, and Arya was able to identify a serious whānau problem that she was sure had directly affected both George and his sister Makere.

The predicament for Makere is an interesting matter as well. At the time I saw her, although I thought that she might have had some spiritual experiences in her life, I wasn't suspecting a spiritual problem. Her Māori CAFS clinician and I had focused on her symptoms of depression and how to address these due to the distress they were causing her. Her seizure-like episodes seemed to be reducing in frequency and intensity by the first few weeks we saw her. We had hoped that by addressing her low mood and the areas of stress in her life, this problem would fade away. It was clear to us that one of the most stressful things for her was the illness George was experiencing. Subsequently, Arya dated the cessation of Makere's pseudoseizures and mood problems to the day of the session with Wiremu, even though Makere didn't attend.

Wiremu

As soon as George came into the staffroom that first time, I could tell that there was a presence there, but this time the presence behind the eyes did not want me to see it. I picked up this female presence—even though he had previously said it sounded deep and masculine, it definitely felt female to me, and very controlling. It was trying to hide and didn't want to be detected by me. It was a creepy thing and I would almost say it felt evil. Some of the stuff it had been putting George through was very unpleasant. Later on, when he was having his convulsion, that felt to me like a clear statement by something other than a human entity—that he was 'hers'. It was a clear indication that she was bent on staying: 'I'm not moving.' I thought: 'You cheeky thing! You're gonna move alright!'

My kuia, my Nanny who came from Tūhoe, never spoke English until she died at 73 years of age. Everything she did was done in karakia. She told me that when something like what George was experiencing happens, there's usually whaiwhaiā: someone or something is usually spiritually pursuing a particular person in order to impose on or punish the person, 'to teach them a lesson'. So this could be a type of curse and it could be put on him by a living person. Sometimes it can happen without the knowledge of the offended party—it's as if their whakapapa has taken over. I would say that this is a very good reason why it's always important to talk mindfully to or about people because you don't know who they are or what they carry. People sometimes say it's not the ones you can see that you ought to worry about—it's the ones you can't see. And very often that unseen someone or something has been a lot more involved in the whānau dynamics further back up the genealogical line. My Nanny used to make a distinction between whaiwhaiā (being pursued spiritually) and mākutu. And she would say that mākutu was about a historic transgression that may have occurred in a previous generation, whereas whaiwhaiā is about a more recent incident when someone has taken offence. There is a saying: 'Ngā hara o ngā tīpuna, ka heke haere mai ki ngā reanga o tēnei wā'—the sins or transgressions of the forefathers will be visited on the generations further down the line. And this whakatauākī is referring to mākutu. However, these effects can be interrupted if the matters are attended to and resolved. And that's where whakawetewete comes in, as I explained to George and Arya in this session. That's the process of forgiving and releasing past unresolved hurts or offences.

So in George's case this entity imposed itself on him; it forced its way in. I would say it was a type of possession that was happening to him. It had his mind. It could create a behaviour in him when it felt like it. That's a possession. That's one kind of mate Māori (Māori sickness). Generally I think that possession is an overused word so I tend not to use it—it's often used for making movies and to push book sales!

When we met up with George and Arya two months after my session with them, I couldn't detect the entity. And that thing can't hide so well that I wouldn't have picked it up if it was really there. I put this down to him being able to do a makeover in his mind. It was about the restoration of his mana. Once it had been explained to him, he had more power to fight back. The more he established his mana, the less this entity had a hold over him. So it had to retreat as it had nothing to hold onto. He was starting to kick it around every day. He was getting stronger. It's not impossible that the entity could've returned if he stopped looking after himself or smoked cannabis again; but I doubted that it would. He stopped his medication within a week or two after our session. So if it was going to take over again, it should have happened in the first month or two.

I liked the way George said he felt it go past, 'Oh, I should know that . . . that was it!' Because it does mean that as he is going along and as he gets stronger, his mind is starting to renew, it's starting to take on board that 'I don't have to accept this', that it's not there anymore.

These kinds of entities will try to deny the young person's improvement and say, 'Nah it hasn't really happened. It hasn't really taken place.' These negative things have been hanging around you and they know what makes you tick and what sets you off. They can be quite aware of those vulnerabilities so that they can exploit your weakness. But with George's renewing of his mind, he was saying, 'Phht, you're out of here!' When we met up two months after the session, George looked to me like he had done a lot of that. He looked blimmin' good!

When I think about George's comments from five years later, I'm not surprised that he could be affected like that by being in close confines with his workmates—because I'm tuned in, too, I can also pick up everybody else's baggage. And if there are any spiritual germs floating around the place, they could attach to him. But he's learning how to discard those germs now, how to protect himself. Some time he'll reach a point where he is much less affected.

As for the pounamu (greenstone) pendant he picked up, every object has a mauri, a life force. And the mauri of that pounamu came from his cousin, who had worn it close to her skin. You could say that the mauri of the pounamu reached out to him and invited him to pick it up. You can read more about this in the next chapter on Caleb, who had a very different experience from picking something up.

There is one more thing I'd like to comment on. Arya talked about both her children being afflicted: not only George but also his sister Makere had been suffering. Makere had been getting depressed, but she had also been getting these same convulsions or fits that George had been getting, though perhaps not so dramatic. I would love to know how a psychiatrist is going to explain that one—two siblings suddenly start having fits within a month of each other! From a spiritual point of view, this can be explained as the same negative entity that must have been impinging on both of them. The cause is connected, as they had both been affected by that raruraru in the family, and they are both susceptible to the unresolved events that had taken place back up in their genealogical line. Interestingly, after our meeting with George, all his sister's fits also went away—and she wasn't even there at the meeting.

How would science explain this? I would guess that the answer to that question is that it would be in the 'too hard' basket. But for me it shows the way things are. For us as Māori, everything is interconnected. I can shake someone's hand and, through doing so, I may see their tīpuna, or I may see something that has taken place. Alternatively, I may see their kidney or their liver or the lung or the heart of the person. I may have a knowing that they are pregnant, even though no one else is aware of this. I'm not saying this to brag about it. It's not even me doing it. If it's shown to me then it must have come from my source for some purpose. To me it just illustrates this awareness that we are whole beings. Everything inside us, around us, below us, and above us is connected.

Notes

1. George's story has been previously published as a case report in a psychiatric journal (Bush & NiaNia, 2012).
2. The extensive use of transcribed interactions from George's session with Wiremu has been included to allow the reader an experience as close as possible to being there.
3. These reflections were prepared from interviews with George and Arya, three months, one year, and five years after Wiremu's intervention session. The interviews were audiotaped, transcribed, and rendered into text by Allister.
4. The medication prescribed was risperidone. Antipsychotic medications are prescribed as a treatment for psychotic symptoms such as hallucinations or delusional beliefs that may be part of a psychotic illness.
5. EIS sees young people who may be having their first experiences of a psychotic illness. However, George's 'voice' was not accompanied by delusions or disorganised thinking or behaviour (except for the seizure-like episodes) or other features of a major psychotic illness, and it was the absence of those factors that led his psychiatrist to consider possible nonpsychotic diagnoses such as dissociation, conversion disorder, or a cultural problem and convinced her to refer him on to our Māori CAF service.
6. This segment of dialogue has been reconstructed from notes that I took of George's comments at the time of this interview. All the details from George and Arya's responses accurately reflect the descriptions they gave in the original interview. All other dialogue in this book is edited transcript of audiorecordings of sessions, unless otherwise stated.
7. Such symptoms, as stated earlier in this chapter, may include delusions (fixed false beliefs not consistent with the person's cultural background and not amenable to reason), disorganised thinking and behaviour, or 'prodromal' symptoms of schizophrenia such as marked and sustained loss of motivation and coping. In George's case, it was true that he felt persecuted by the voice; however, this wasn't a delusion as his response seemed reasonable given what the voice had been telling him.

References

Arseneault, L., Cannon, M., Poulton, R., Murray, R., Caspi, A. & Moffitt, T.E. (2002) 'Cannabis use in adolescence and risk for adult psychosis: Longitudinal prospective study'. *British Medical Journal* 325: 1212–13.

Bodde, N.M.G., Brooks, J.L., Baker, G.A., Boon, P.A.J.M., Hendriksen, J.G.M., Mulder, O.G. & Aldenkamp, A.P. (2009) 'Psychogenic non-epileptic seizures—Definition, etiology, treatment and prognostic issues: A critical review'. *Seizure* 18: 543–53.

Bush, A. & NiaNia, W. (2012) 'Voice hearing and pseudoseizures in a Māori teenager: An example of mate Māori and Māori traditional healing'. *Australasian Psychiatry* 20: 348–51.

Gabbard, G. (2005) *Psychodynamic psychiatry in clinical practice* (4th edn). American Psychiatric Publishing, Arlington.

Sadock, B.J. & Sadock, V.A. (2005) *Kaplan and Sadock's comprehensive textbook of psychiatry* (8th edn). Lippincott Williams & Wilkins, New York.

5

THE LESSON

This chapter describes the story of Caleb, a 17-year-old Cook Islands and New Zealand Māori young man who had grown up in the care of his Cook Islands maternal grandparents. His dramatic experience, which might appear from a psychiatric point of view to be a kind of psychotic symptom, can also be understood from a Māori perspective as a form of mate Māori (Māori sickness). In the second part of the chapter, Allister, Wiremu, and Caleb offer three perspectives on Caleb's story and experiences. First, Allister provides a psychiatric viewpoint. Second, Wiremu outlines his views about these puzzling phenomena and shows how an understanding of concepts such as mauri (life force) and tapu (that which is sacred or forbidden) can help illuminate this territory from the spectrum of Māori worldviews. Finally, Caleb reflects back on his own experience from hindsight seven years later.

Allister

Introducing Caleb

As Caleb prepared to leave his house that morning, he had no inkling of how that day would turn out. His grandparents had already gone to work, leaving him behind on his own. He had slept in again. As he pulled his school uniform on, Caleb wondered vaguely if there was some homework that he had overlooked. He was already running late and knew he had no time for breakfast. He walked around the living room, gathering his things. Slinging his school bag over his shoulder, Caleb opened the front door and walked quickly down the path, brushing his hair out of his eyes. Suddenly he stopped. There in front of him was a startling vision. Just beyond his front gate he saw a large Māori warrior blocking his path. This terrifying figure was naked from the waist up and towering over Caleb. He was a very dark-looking Māori man with long, jet-black, wavy hair and a facial moko (tattoo) that covered only the right side of his face. He spoke rapidly and fiercely at Caleb in Māori. He was clearly enraged and was brandishing a long taiaha (spear-shaped weapon), waving it threateningly towards Caleb and banging it on the ground in an intimidating manner. Horrified, Caleb fled back inside the house.

He flung himself down on the couch in the living room and turned on the TV and the stereo. His hands were trembling. He could feel his heart pounding in his chest. His mind was whirling. He tried to distract himself by focusing on the infomercial on the TV screen. 'What the hell was that?' he wondered. After some minutes of staring at the TV screen his heart wasn't racing quite so much. He tried to think about his next step: he was already late for school, and he knew it wouldn't take much for his English teacher to give him another detention for tardiness. Was his mind playing a trick on him? Maybe it was some weird thing he'd imagined. He took a deep breath and braced himself. He grabbed his bag and headed out the door again.

Just beyond the gate the apparition was still there. The figure seemed just as enraged as at their earlier encounter. Caleb beat a retreat back inside again. He had no idea what this thing was but it certainly freaked him out. He could tell it wasn't a real flesh-and-blood person because the image he could see was suspended there above the ground. But it was very loud and staunch. What did this warrior want with him? The figure had some kind of olden-day material around his waist. He sure was enraged about something. Caleb was fairly certain that the figure was yelling at him in Māori, as he was studying Māori at school. His grandparents were native Cook Islands Māori speakers, and he could distinguish the language of this warrior's wrath from his grandparents' vernacular.

After hiding for another 10 minutes, Caleb knew he had to do something. He headed out the door yet again. The warrior remained just beyond their gate, barring his way to the bus stop. This time Caleb pulled his hoodie down over his face, put his head down, bolted out the gate, and ran for half a block until he was far enough away from his house to dare to pause for breath. He couldn't see the warrior now. His chest was heaving as he caught his breath and his heart was pounding again. He was still feeling quite panicky when he arrived at school.

Over the next two weeks the same figure reappeared to him most mornings at the same time and in the same place. He also saw it once outside his school. By now he would break out in a cold sweat merely at the thought of leaving for school in the mornings. Some days he would become terror-stricken at school when he thought about the figure. At these times his heart would start to race so much that he found it hard to catch his breath. He would feel dizzy, with a tightening around his head and tingling and numbness in his legs and feet.

When one of his teachers noticed his obvious discomfort, he was referred to the school guidance counsellor. At first he didn't want to tell her about his experience, as he feared she would think he was crazy, but at last he confided in her. Once he had explained his experience to her in some detail, she went away and spoke to a colleague. She was concerned that he was experiencing some kind of hallucination and psychosis. She returned and recommended she send a referral to the Early Intervention Service (EIS) for an urgent assessment.

Meanwhile, Caleb's te reo Māori teacher at the college heard about his experience. Believing that this could represent some kind of mate Māori phenomenon, she asked Caleb for his permission to arrange for a tohunga—a Māori traditional healer—to meet with him at school. The next day, during his Māori class, his teacher asked him to step next door into the marae. There she introduced him to the Māori elder she had invited to the school to meet with him. She explained that he was a tohunga and could help him.

The tohunga didn't speak directly to Caleb. It was raining outside, and the tohunga went out for a while and collected some of the rainwater in a bowl. When he returned he stood before Caleb and recited a karakia in Māori. As he did so he picked up handfuls of the water, which he tossed over Caleb. He then took Caleb out into the rain and resumed the karakia. After this he left. Caleb was mystified by this process.

However, he was surprised and very relieved the next morning to discover that the apparition had gone. Despite its disappearance, it was hard to get it out of his mind, and each morning he remained very apprehensive as he was preparing to leave for school. At school his episodes of panic persisted.

At the time of his first appointment with the EIS clinicians, Caleb recounted his experiences in some detail. It was now about a week since he had seen the tohunga, and the visions of the warrior had not returned. The EIS team concluded that it was unlikely that he had a major psychotic illness, but they wondered about a drug-related problem or a cultural problem in addition to his anxiety symptoms. They recommended to Caleb that he be referred on to the Māori Child, Adolescent and Family Service (Māori CAFS) team.

At his first appointment with the Māori CAFS team, he met with Wiremu. During this interview Caleb admitted to a direct query that three weeks before the first appearance of the apparition he had found a large, beautiful pounamu (greenstone) pendant on the road and had put it around his neck. Over the next few days he had become aware of a strange feeling that he couldn't explain—that he was being watched by some disapproving presence. However, he dismissed this as perhaps his guilty conscience and defiantly carried on wearing the pendant.

Caleb's father was Māori, but had moved away to another city early in Caleb's life, so Caleb had grown up with his Cook Islands maternal grandparents. Caleb had only seen his father very infrequently. Caleb did not report using marijuana or other illicit substances in the weeks leading up to the appearance of the mysterious apparition. He hadn't suffered from depression or any major anxiety problem before the morning the apparition first appeared, and there wasn't anyone he knew of in his extended family with major problems like these. He was not experiencing any other psychotic symptoms apart from the visions of the figure, who he could hear yelling at him. He did say that for some months he had been arguing more with his grandparents; however, he didn't consider this to be different from what his mates of the same age were going through with their parents.

Wiremu was convinced that the information about the pounamu was the key to understanding this cultural puzzle. Wiremu advised Caleb to dispose of the pounamu and asked if he could karakia for him to seek a blessing for this process. He explained to Caleb about Māori concepts of mana, mauri, and tapu so that Caleb could understand what had happened and how this made sense from the point of view of te ao Māori (the Māori world). He explained that it was akin to a spiritual germ that he had caught when he picked up the piece of pounamu: this pounamu must have previously belonged to a Māori person with enough mana and mauri that an ancestor of that person had objected strongly to Caleb wearing it around his own neck. This action on Caleb's part had, unbeknownst to him, constituted a breach of tapu. The karakia from the tohunga had the effect of purifying the situation, but the initial breach of tapu had to be put right for the matter to be properly resolved.

After these matters were explained to Caleb, and when the apparition failed to return, his panic symptoms gradually subsided. When I had an opportunity to meet with Caleb two weeks after he had seen Wiremu, he had no further evidence of any psychotic symptoms. His anxiety symptoms were also much improved. He told me that he was happy with the explanation that Wiremu had given him, as it made sense to him from his Cook Islands upbringing with his grandparents but also what he had learnt from his New Zealand Māori side.

Making Sense of Caleb's Experience from a Western Psychiatry Viewpoint

From a psychiatric perspective, it is not easy to make sense of the scenario that Caleb was faced with prior to the intervention of the tohunga. It is uncommon for people to have a psychotic experience in which the auditory and visual stimuli are in synchrony. Furthermore, how do we make sense of Caleb hearing a voice yelling at him in Māori when the languages he is most familiar with are English and Cook Islands Māori? And why would these experiences cease altogether after the brief intervention from the tohunga?

From a Western secular viewpoint, one explanation could be that perhaps there was a powerful placebo effect from the ritual carried out by the tohunga, even if Caleb didn't understand or have strong faith in the process. However, severe psychotic symptoms aren't generally thought to be so susceptible to the power of suggestion. Often, in psychiatry, unusual experiences like this can be attributed to hallucinations caused by the use of drugs such as cannabis or hallucinogens; but Caleb didn't report using any substances in the weeks leading up to the onset of his vivid experiences, and he was frightened enough by the experiences that he said he would gladly have owned up to using a substance if that could have explained the problem.

Psychotic illnesses like schizophrenia can cause severe and frightening hallucinations. However, schizophrenia is associated with other problems such as withdrawing from friends, disorganised thinking and behaviour, and delusions or false beliefs—for example, that one is being persecuted by others. Although he was very anxious about his experience, Caleb did not have any of these other symptoms of psychosis.

From a Western mental health viewpoint, the information about the pounamu is irrelevant. From the viewpoint of te ao Māori, it is an important clue to the cause of the problem. In the next section Wiremu outlines in more detail how this scenario could be understood from within the spectrum of Māori worldviews.

Wiremu

Within te ao Māori, it is commonly accepted that we are spiritual beings first and foremost. It's important to understand that if you want to make sense of Caleb's experience. The next point is that everything has a mauri, which is like the energy or life force of a person. But if something like a piece of pounamu or a bone carving is worn close to your skin for a long time, it will pick up your mauri and, by doing so, the pounamu begins to have a mauri of its own. And so this young fella picked up a taonga, a precious object—a piece of pounamu belonging to someone else. It had their mauri inherent in it. The Māori warrior yelling at him is likely to be a kēhua or spirit, some ancestor of the person whose taonga it was. Caleb identified him as looking like a Māori and said he had a kind of cloth around his waist. In the old days that would have been a rāpaki covering that part of the body. And this warrior is admonishing him, telling him off and giving him a hard time. But he's not grabbing him or anything. He's not actually hurting him, but rather just giving him a fright.

And because it's a spiritual problem, it can be remedied with a spiritual solution. Once Caleb had the karakia with that tohunga and carefully disposed of the other person's taonga in the right way, then the problem disappears. Except that he is still really freaking out about it for a while longer—but the more he understands about it, the more that anxiety settles down. That's why I always try to explain to young fellas like Caleb about what is going on so they can understand.

And so an interesting question here is: Was this a psychotic episode or was it a Māori-related experience? My money is on the Māori-related experience. Let me explain more about mauri and tapu.

Mauri

As I said before, if you pick up someone's taonga, it has their mauri in it, so really it has its own mauri—the mauri of that person has transferred onto that object. Whether it's a bone piece, mere (club), or taiaha, it holds that person's mauri because it's been intimate to that person. So the energy or life force has been transferred onto the object. It's like your violin, Allister. People can pick it up, but they'll never play it the same way as you do, because your mauri is in that instrument. It's like someone picking up some famous tennis player's racquet. It has that player's mauri in it, so, unless it was given to them, it will cause them, for example, to be a bad player. If you pick up someone's taonga and put it on without their permission or blessing, this could cause you to have all sorts of experiences similar to those of Caleb. So we would always be very careful about that.

Tapu

An example of tapu in te ao Māori is that it would be tapu, or forbidden, to pick up and wear clothing from some dead person. That would be a breach of tapu. And there would be some kind of consequence for breaching that tapu, even if you were innocent of any knowledge of the owner. It's not just something people think might happen, it does happen. It has happened to a lot of people. If you took clothing from a deceased person, usually illness would follow. Someone would get sick, someone would die—and I mean, we all die, but they would die in some strange way. So if someone directly related to you dies and you might have lent their clothes to someone in that genealogical line, then that could very well be the explanation for a person in the same genealogical line getting sick. And again, because this is a spiritual problem, it requires a spiritual solution to remedy it.

I would say that tapu is something that we believe is inherent from God or Io. Each person has a tapu of their own. For example, I would consider that you're tapu, and so in respect of that I'd try not to get into your space because that's tapu, that's yours—yours alone. It is the same as respecting someone with mana, say, a doctor. A doctor has mana from a Māori perspective because they use their skill and knowledge to help people get well. In the old days there was a tapu on you as a doctor that people gave a lot of respect to: you could probably leave the door to your house open and no one would enter because it was tapu. And it belonged to you, and to tramp on that meant that there were going to be repercussions.

I'll give you an example that relates to tikanga. At a pōwhiri (ceremonial welcome) or tangihanga (bereavement ritual) especially, there is a tapu on the people, the manuhiri, who have never been there before. They are called waewae tapu because they have never trodden on that place before. And at a tangi, the tūpāpaku, or dead person, also carries an amount of tapu. There are protocols for protecting the living from this tapu that need to be strictly followed. In general we consider that when you come across the dead, they have a tapu that's not conducive to our well-being as a living person. According to our tikanga we have to make sure that we don't encroach on or cross these spiritual boundaries, either knowingly or unknowingly, or else ill fortune will fall on us.

You could compare it to the medical idea of germs. From a medical perspective you would treat a dead body carefully because you could pick up some bacteria that may be harmful to you, and so the body needs to be treated in a certain way such as embalming. Of course, respect for tapu will also protect you from these physical germs, and that's helpful. But there is a spiritual role for tapu as well: it helps us avoid picking up unwanted spiritual germs that can definitely negatively affect your wairua and well-being.

The other side of tapu is the noa (free from tapu) part. You see this in the tikanga of a pōwhiri where everything is tapu during the karanga (calling people onto the marae) and the whaikōrero or speeches, until you get to the hongi[1] and the actual physical contact—and then all that is made noa by having the hākari (sharing of food) afterwards. Sitting down to eat together transforms a tapu process into noa. And that makes it safe from a spiritual point of view. And that process has to be done.

In Chapter 2 I talked about one of our ancestors, Tānenuiārangi, who ascended into the heavenly realms and acquired three kete, or baskets, of knowledge that pertain to us as human beings. After he acquired these kete, he planted them into Papatūānuku, and out of that came us as humans. We had our own belief systems well before we had the Christian influence. It's interesting for me how new belief systems can come and how they can add on to the older belief systems that were handed down from generation to generation. Science is an example that I find really interesting. Science can't disprove that there is a spirit. Scientists can raise doubts about certain claims and even try to disprove certain hypotheses about the nature of things, but science can't disprove there is a spirit. It can only prove there is.

Here we have an example with Caleb in which psychiatry as a scientific discipline is having a hard time trying to explain his experience. For me, in that case it makes sense to look for another explanation from a different belief system that might help us make sense of what is going on. And in this case you have to look into the wairua side to find the cause.

Caleb Looks Back

I'm 24 years old now and it's more than seven years ago that this all happened to me. Although mostly I would prefer not to think about it, many aspects of it are still very vivid for me. I can very clearly remember how the warrior looked. His face was striking. I'm a very visual person. After I ran inside, as well as freaking out, I was puzzled about why he only had the moko on the right half of his face. I'd never seen that before, and it seemed uncomfortably strange. A year ago, after talking to Allister about this chapter, I spoke to a friend of mine. She suggested that perhaps the appearance of his moko was somehow a reflection of the two sides of my family: only half of my genealogy is New Zealand Māori. Somehow that made sense to me.

I can also very clearly remember meeting the tohunga. When I was pulled out of my class and into the marae, I didn't know what was going on. I remember he found the bowl and put rainwater in it and while he said the karakia he splashed the water from the bowl over me. At that point I was standing in the doorway of the marae. It was raining and he indicated that he wanted to me to stand outside in the rain, and he repeated the karakia and made me stand out there for 15 to 20 minutes. Then I remember returning and sitting down and he said something else in Māori. My teacher came back in and they were talking and it was pretty much over. I didn't know if it had worked. I didn't know what to make of it, as I wasn't told anything.

Some time later my counsellor came to see me and said that there was an appointment for me with the Māori mental health service. And I'm not going to lie: I didn't want to meet with them at the time. I'm not good with meeting a lot of new people. But although I was reluctant I was taken into Te Whare Mārie and introduced to Wiremu. It helped me meeting an elder who wasn't speaking only in Māori. He was a down-to-earth guy and he just made me feel really relaxed and at home. I explained to him about the pounamu and that I'd put it on and then everything else that had happened as a consequence of that. Wiremu helped me make sense of everything that had happened. He talked me through tapu and Māori customs and explained to me why I should have left the pounamu where I had found it. That explanation provided me with a reason for the figure appearing to me and barring my way and why I was so afraid of it. Being able to make sense of it like that helped me find some kind of closure. I didn't feel so crazy anymore. Because that's how I felt while it was happening. In the school marae, I had felt very uncomfortable with the whole thing because I had no idea what was going on. I just went with it because I was getting so hacked off that whenever I tried to go to school, I was panicking and hyperventilating.

Before the first time I saw the warrior, I never had a problem with anxiety, and it's not a usual problem in my family. But that experience shook me up so badly that I kept having panic episodes for some months, even after Wiremu explained it all to me. It took me quite a while to deal with it. However, these days things are much better, and I haven't had problems like that for a long time. I think it's important for young people to have an explanation about these kinds of spiritual things because if they can have the right people to talk to, then they can avoid going down the wrong path and ending up needing drugs to try to get rid of it.

For me this was a really literal and dramatic lesson about tapu and about what not to do and what not to touch with regard to Māori customs. I will never forget it as long as I live.

Note

1. The exchange of breath, representing the sharing of mauri, that takes place when two people press their noses together (Moon, 2003).

Reference

Moon, P. (2003) *Tohunga Hohepa Kereopa*. David Ling Publishing, Auckland.

6

'I WILL NOT LEAVE MY BABY BEHIND'

This chapter describes the story of a 10-year-old Cook Islands girl named Moana[1] told from three different perspectives. It begins with an outline of the family predicament and background context, and then a description of the session with the family narrated by Allister. The next section is told from the perspective of Wiremu. The final voice is that of Tere, Moana's mother. Each narration brings a different perspective, and together they illuminate a multidimensional family therapy process that extends beyond immediate and living family members and takes account of genealogical and intergenerational influences.

Allister

Family Situation

Tere rang to refer her daughter Moana to our Pasifika Child, Adolescent and Family Service (Health Pasifika CAFS) with an unusual but intriguing request. She said that she would like our urgent help with her daughter, but insisted on a cultural focus rather than purely a mental health assessment. Given that she was convinced her daughter's difficulties were related to a cultural problem, she wondered if we might provide this. Everyone in the family was becoming very distressed about Moana's strange and disturbed behaviour, which only occurred at night.

We met urgently with Moana and her mother, her nine-year-old sister Melanie, and her four-year-old brother. Tere explained that eight weeks before our meeting, she and her new husband William had returned from their honeymoon in the Cook Islands, during which time the three children had stayed at home with their grandmother. This had been Tere's first visit back to her ancestral home in the Cook Islands since leaving there and emigrating to Aotearoa (New Zealand) at the age of 12. Two weeks after their return, Moana started waking up before midnight agitated, angry, and then strangely distant and withdrawn. Sometimes her agitated behaviour went on for several hours during the night and it was very frightening for the family. At times Moana would become so enraged, she would lash out at her mother and stepfather, and she showed surprising strength for her age and size when they tried to restrain her. Tere and her husband talked about a 'disturbing look' that indicated to them that she had had 'a total personality change'. Although previously she could sometimes be strong willed, she was usually respectful and helpful and took her responsibilities as the eldest sibling seriously.

During several of these episodes Moana had spoken in the ancestral dialect of her mother's family, using vocabulary and ancestral names for particular family members that her mother believed that she couldn't possibly know. One night Moana's grandmother encouraged Tere to talk to an agitated Moana in their ancestral dialect. Tere asked her, 'Who are you? What do you want?' Moana spat at her mother and then responded angrily: 'Kāre au e akaruke i tāku pēpe, kā tākinokino ia e kōtou!' (I will not leave my baby behind because you people will hurt her).

At other times Moana said she could see shadows and faces in the corner of her bedroom, and one night she told of seeing an old lady with long grey hair and a walking stick in the same corner. Moana's anxiety, sleep disturbance, and episodes of agitated behaviour persisted in the weeks leading up to our first meeting, and her mother and stepfather were becoming exhausted.

Suspecting a spiritual problem, Tere sought assistance from their church pastor, who had a Pacific background. He blessed Moana, her family, and their house. For a few days there was an improvement in Moana's disturbed nocturnal behaviour, but then it worsened again. Tere consulted local New Zealand Māori kaumātua, who arrived the same night as the pastor and encouraged her to continue with the pastor. Tere also consulted her mother and other senior family members, who supported her view that this was a cultural problem known as maki tūpāpaku.[2] But no matter what, Moana's nocturnal distress and agitation did not let up. Tere was reluctant to seek help from a mental health service, as she feared that her daughter's problem could be misdiagnosed as a mental health disorder. However, eventually her desperation reached such a point that she decided to do so.

Our child mental health service was set up to address the mental health needs of Pacific children, young people, and their families in our local area in Aotearoa (Bush et al., 2009). Local referrers to the service are generally aware that we put a strong emphasis on Pasifika cultural values in our interactions with families. Most of our staff are of Pacific descent, and we have a Samoan cultural consultant, Fa'amausili Chapman, who is a matai (titled elder) and is available to join us in our meetings with families.

Background Family Context

Matters had been difficult for some time between Tere and John, her ex-husband and Moana's father. Their separation in Moana's preschool years became increasingly acrimonious as they waged a legal battle over custody of Moana and her sister. Tere spoke wistfully about the warm and mutually affectionate relationship that she had always enjoyed with Moana. She willingly acknowledged that it had been a stressful time leading up to her recent wedding and wondered if she had been so distracted that she had lost touch with Moana.

From my psychiatric viewpoint, there was no suggestion of previous physical or sexual trauma, although Moana had witnessed conflict between her parents in her preschool years. Her mother recalled Moana's first year of life as difficult, but did not think she had been depressed. There was no psychosis reported in the family. Moana had no previous epilepsy or other medical problems and did not seem depressed. She was, however, anxious about things in general and most worried at night, but at a loss to explain the source of her worry. Other than the faces and shadows she saw, Moana had no other symptoms suggesting psychosis. She had no recall of the nocturnal events that Tere and her husband were reporting.

When I met with John, he didn't report similar episodes when Moana stayed with him. However, of late these visits had been infrequent because of Tere's concerns about Moana.

At this point in the first meetings with the family, I was puzzled about Moana's experiences and symptoms. They didn't fit into a recognised diagnostic category. Some elements resembled a psychotic process, or possibly a dissociative process as a result of trauma. However, the most obvious stress Moana was under was the ongoing acrimony and lack of communication between her mother and father. This could easily have been exacerbated during the preparations for Tere's wedding, and it seemed the most likely systemic explanation for her distress. Still, this did not account for Tere's description of Moana's utterances in her ancestral dialect in the most conflicted moments—which I found intriguing.

Through my contact with colleagues from the Family Centre, Lower Hutt (Waldegrave et al., 2003) and my work in Māori and Pacific indigenous services, Tere's description reminded me of accounts of rare instances of people who had been thought by family members to be 'possessed'. I was struck by Tere's conviction that Moana was suffering from a cultural problem and her labelling this problem as 'possession'. I wanted to understand how Tere had come to this conclusion in order to work with her to unravel this puzzle and hopefully find some relief for Moana and the family.

Tere's Early Experiences

Tere was born in Aotearoa (New Zealand), but in her infancy returned to her ancestral home in the Cook Islands.[3] From her infancy until she was eight years old, Tere was cared for primarily by her Nana (grandmother) as well as her Vouvou (great-great-grandmother), the ta'unga (Cook Islands traditional healer) of the local community, who was by then in her nineties. Tere had been sent to live with her Vouvou because she was the eldest child in her generation, just as her mother and grandmother had been before her. During these formative years, Tere was almost always in the presence of this elderly matriarch, who conversed with Tere in their ancestral tongue and instructed her about traditional understandings regarding the ancestors and their relationships to spirituality. She gave priority to her Christianity by insisting that 'God is more powerful than spirits' and is 'the best source of strength' when faced with spiritual problems.

Tere's Vouvou died when Tere was eight, after a fortnight during which she was bedridden. Two nights before she died she appeared, to everyone's astonishment, at two in the morning, dressed and outside her house with a bundle of clothes. She was addressing a number of deceased ancestors: 'Te tiaki nei au i tāku pēpe, ko māua kā ano atu ei' (I'm waiting for my baby girl, we're coming together). The 'girl' she was referring to was assumed to be Tere. She then announced to the adults present: 'Kāre au e akaruke i tāku pēpe, kā tākinokino ia e kōtou!'

Several years after her great-great-grandmother's death, Tere went to live with her mother in Aotearoa. She returned to the Cook Islands, although not to her ancestral home, in her late teens with her parents, who were immersed in considerable conflict with each other. One night Tere awoke in the early hours agitated and angry, although she had very little recollection of that the next day. Her family reported it took five able-bodied adults to restrain her, and she was shouting: 'Kāre au e akaruke i tāku pēpe, kā tākinokino ia e kōtou!' The adults present had no doubt these words not only sounded like her great-great-grandmother, but, in fact, were her speaking through Tere. Immediately after, Tere called out to her mother, this time in English: 'Mum, please don't let me go!'

Tere recalled one other episode similar to this when she was in her early twenties, during a time when she was distressed about her relationship with John.

After hearing Tere's life story, I was convinced that there was more to this than a psychiatric perspective could hope to unravel. We all agreed that we needed cultural expertise to help us make sense of it and to seek an appropriate resolution—ideally a traditional healer from their Cook Islands culture and community. However, the family had already exhausted their own contacts. At our service at that time we did not know of any Cook Islands traditional healers in our local community.

In the absence of such contacts, I tentatively suggested a consultation with my colleague Wiremu. I explained that I had worked closely with Wiremu over a five-year period and trusted his judgement on such matters. I said that he had frequently been able to help families with spiritual problems, often in surprising ways. I raised with them a major doubt that I had, which was that they were from a Cook Islands background, whereas Wiremu is New Zealand Māori.

Tere said she was comfortable to consult a practitioner from a New Zealand Māori background because of the close genealogical connections between their cultures. Tere and her husband and Moana's father John immediately accepted my proposal of a consultation with Wiremu.

Family Healing Intervention

I could feel the tension in the room as we commenced our meeting with the family. Tere was seated next to her husband, William, with Moana on her other side. On the opposite side of the room Moana's father John sat next to Moana's sister Melanie. I noticed that Wiremu had placed himself right next to John, and after a brief moment he made a light-hearted comment and reached out and placed a friendly hand on his shoulder; I could see that John relaxed a little after that.

Our Pacific cultural consultant, Fa'amausili, mindful of the Christian affiliations of many Pacific families, sought the family's permission to begin the session with a prayer. When they readily agreed, he offered a prayer and then welcomed everyone and suggested that we have a round of introductions. Wiremu was the last to introduce himself, and he described his role as a cultural therapist. He said that although he did not consider himself to be an expert, especially on Cook Islands cultural matters, he hoped he would be able to offer something helpful for the family. He then asked if I would say a few words about the family's concerns so that he could understand more about their situation. I thanked everyone for coming and acknowledged that it was a sign of Tere and John's commitment to Moana that they both chose to attend, despite their differences. Then I summarised their concerns about Moana—the times when she would be angry, upset, and unable to sleep and yet she couldn't remember anything about it the next day. I spoke of Tere's concern that there could be a cultural or spiritual problem behind these matters, and mentioned that we were meeting Wiremu in the hope that he might be able to help us all understand this better and perhaps resolve the matter.

Right before the meeting I had briefed Wiremu, explaining who was in the family and that Tere was wondering if Moana was suffering from some kind of 'possession'. I told him that Tere and John, Moana's birth father, had separated some years before and that things might be tense between them, especially as her new husband was there as well, but in spite of this they had agreed to meet together on behalf of Moana. This was the only information that Wiremu had when he first stepped into the room.

After Wiremu exchanged some light-hearted words with Moana and Melanie and their brother left the room to look for toys in the waiting area, Wiremu asked for an opportunity to speak with the adults on their own. I helped the girls find some toys, and they entertained their younger brother in an adjacent room next to the reception area.

Wiremu then addressed John, Tere, and William. He spoke about a feeling of anxiety that he had picked up in his chest area. He said that he had sensed whom he was supposed to be meeting immediately upon setting foot into the room. To make his point, he gestured to where Moana had been sitting. He said that he believed that the anxiety he was picking up was from Moana. At this point Tere, who I had noticed was looking very tense and uncertain, asked Wiremu, 'Did you pick up anything around Moana?' Wiremu responded, 'There is a presence here which looked at me and then withdrew.' Looking intently at Wiremu, Tere then asked him: 'Can you tell what gender?' Instead of a direct reply to her inquiry, Wiremu met her searching gaze and responded carefully, 'Let me answer that by asking you: How did you get on with your grandmother?'

This response both shocked and reassured her. It was at this point that there was a marked change in Tere's demeanour. Her shoulders relaxed, and she spoke to Wiremu about her concerns about Moana and the difficulties over the previous weeks. I sensed that she had accepted something implicit in Wiremu's query and that this had reassured her that she could trust him. Tere talked without any restraint about her conviction that there was something cultural that was interfering with Moana's well-being. She wondered if it might be some local spiritual matter—perhaps Moana had accidentally breached a New Zealand Māori tapu in the area where they lived. Or could it have arisen from her recent visit to her ancestral home in the Cook Islands? Tere explained that she had her own experiences of 'cultural issues' from her earlier years. Then she raised a question about demonic possession.

Wiremu responded to this question by saying:

> Sometimes we are influenced by our Christian beliefs to think that there is a demonic presence or a demonic possession, and that most things that are unexplainable are demonic. However, from the point of view of our tīpuna (ancestors), there are many other explanations. Sometimes the ancestors use these ways to send a message to the living. The message may be to sound the alarm or to alert us to a problem. It may be a wake-up call from the other side.

Wiremu explained that he had a strong feeling that the old lady he could see was giving the family a message that if the girl wasn't looked after, then she would come and take her. He explained that from a New Zealand Māori point of view, 'the actions of the generation before and the generation before that come down upon the younger generation' and so, often, answers can been found in the whakapapa, in problems that occurred between people, or breaches of tapu in previous generations.

Wiremu now asked more questions about both sides of the family. He conversed with Tere and at the same time, when he referred either directly or indirectly to John in the conversation, he would rest a supportive hand on John's shoulder. John remained silent, but when Wiremu directed a question to him, he spoke of Moana's recent anxiety and difficulty sleeping.

Soon after this Wiremu addressed his concern about the rift between Tere and John. The following transcript illustrates how he approached this matter. As we join the conversation, Tere is speaking about her intuitive awareness about when things aren't going well for Moana, even if she is away from Tere's presence.

Tere: I don't know if it's a gift or something that has been passed on. I'm probably still trying to find answers, especially when they are away with him [the girls' father John] . . . I'm having either anxiety or chest pains or something like that. But as I'm getting older I'm acknowledging . . . Is it a gift or is it a mother's connection to their children? I don't know.

Wiremu: (speaking softly, gently but firmly) There will always be a mother's connection to their children. Tere, I'm just making an observation here. You know how we were talking about bringing closure so that unresolved issues from past generations don't get passed on to the children. I notice that you refer to John as 'him' a lot. Part of the closure is saying 'John'. That's starting the healing. You take that first step, something spiritually will happen. Because, I've been noticing right throughout the whole meeting, it's 'him' or 'he' or 'his' when you are talking about John. Sorry for making that observation.

Tere: No that's . . . Yeah . . .

Wiremu: I'm just pointing that out. Because I'm talking about bringing about a closure, bringing about something that's good for the kids. So the first thing is, this gentleman over here has a name. (indicating John) If you want to see the benefits or that spiritual shift in the children, then you need to take that first step.

Tere: Oh no, thank you for bringing that up, because that was one of the things I did in my therapy a couple of years ago. See, without even noticing that I'm . . . yeah, thank you for . . . yeah . . . (laughing)

Wiremu: You know you are absolutely in charge of this, you can tell me to shut up! (laughing)

Tere: It's alright.

William: She's says that about me, too.

Wiremu: About 'him'? (laughing)

William: I'm her husband but she calls me 'him'! (general laughter)

Wiremu: (laughing) Yeah and that's a good thing. Each and every one of us in this room has a gift. We all have gifts. And I would say you have a gift and Moana has also got a gift. And I haven't picked up any sort of evil intent on the part of the old people. Actually, I would say there is a group of tīpuna who have a strong motivation to bring it right for the family. And so I put that down as them calling out, hey, this is

> a . . . what do you call it, not a warning, a wake-up call. And one of the ways to start is saying his name.

Wiremu explained that he had come to the conclusion that the rift that the tīpuna were protesting about was the problem between the parents. He said that it was necessary for the well-being of Moana and the other children that the adults find some way to reconcile their differences.

Initially Tere didn't respond to this, but Wiremu came back to it. I noticed he did so with a lot of warmth and aroha (love), but also clarity. At this point, Tere seemed to soften. She paused for some moments. Then she turned and looked directly at her ex-husband John and spoke to him, solemnly uttering each word. She began: 'I am going to pretend that we are the only two people in this room.' For the first time in the meeting she used John's name. She acknowledged that this was the first time they had been in a room together for more than three years. She spoke about matters that had caused pain between them. At this point she paused and seemed to hesitate.

After looking at Wiremu, Tere turned to John once more and apologised for the hurtful things she had said over the years. She spoke about a number of matters that she believed may have brought pain to John, and she asked if he would forgive her.

Then it was John's turn to speak. He acknowledged Tere in their mother tongue. Similarly, he spoke about times when he had become very angry. He also apologised for times when he had done something that caused pain to her. He said that he did forgive her and wanted to find a way to improve things for the sake of their children. In addition, he apologised to Tere's new husband William for any offence he may have caused him. By this time tears were falling down Tere's cheeks. As she wiped them away I noticed tenderness in John's eyes when he looked at her, replacing the uncompromising look I had seen earlier in the session. When their eyes met I sensed that they had both allowed the bitterness and resentment they had been holding on to for a long time to be released. The tension so evident at the beginning of the session had lifted.

Wiremu acknowledged what had been shared and the courage it had taken from all parties. In the pause that followed, Tere's son burst into the room with a picture he had drawn for his mum and dad to look at. While Tere and William admired the picture, I left the room to check on his sisters. The session was nearing the end of the allotted time, and Wiremu knew that it would be important to whakanoa (make free from tapu) the process of reconciliation. He invited the adults present to shake hands or embrace one another, if they felt comfortable to do so. He then embraced each of the three parents in turn, and they embraced each other.

After the children returned, I noticed that they looked more relaxed. I asked Wiremu if he wanted to say a karakia at this point, and he said that it wasn't necessary. He mentioned that he could see that there had been a change and that this was enough for now. I proposed that we explain to the children something about what had happened in the room in their absence, and Wiremu suggested I do that. I proceeded to explain that Wiremu had said that there were some ancestors in the family who were concerned, wanting to help the family, and who wanted the adults to sort out some things, so Wiremu had been encouraging Moana and Melanie's mother and father to let go of some of the hurt from the past.

At this point Wiremu departed and I arranged another appointment time with Tere and Moana. However, the parents and stepfather asked if they could spend some more time talking over matters they needed to sort out that had been unresolved over the last few years. This took another two hours. The children had some lunch and then played together in my office. There was lightness in Moana's countenance as she joked with Melanie and looked after her brother.

When I phoned Tere to check on progress the next week, she said that from the time of the session with Wiremu there had been a very marked change in Moana. She seemed happy and there were no more concerns about her behaviour at night. She was no longer anxious about going off to sleep. Weeks later when we met, Moana was well and there were no more reports of agitated behaviour or any of the other nighttime behaviour that had been so worrying and perplexing for her family. Tere described Moana as back to her normal self. Two years later Moana was still well and thriving.

Wiremu

When I entered the room to meet this family for the first time, my attention was instantly drawn to one particular young lass (Moana), and I immediately recognised which one of the two girls I was supposed to meet. When I observed her more closely, there was a spiritual presence that showed itself to me and then withdrew. I detected an old lady who appeared to be within Moana, a presence there that others couldn't see. The old lady was loving, but she was also stern, like a disciplinarian kind of kuia. When I mentioned the presence, Tere asked me what gender, and I replied, 'How did you get on with your grandmother?'

Well, the kuia showed herself again to me, and I noticed that there were several gentlemen in the background. One was solidly built and round, like myself, with a yellow T-shirt or singlet on. He had a pleasant face and very short hair. He was seated. And standing next to him was an older man with a beard that had been left to grow wild, and he had longish hair with grey streaks. It looked like a discussion was taking place. It felt like it was in a village setting, perhaps from Tere and John's home. They were concerned, but at the same time I could tell that they were really supportive of what was taking place. Their wish seemed to be that whatever was happening to Moana would be brought to a halt with reconciliation.

By this time I'd asked the children to leave the room. I did this because I was concerned that some of the talk about supernatural things might be scary for the children. And I was already confident that the main problem that the tīpuna were protesting about was the raruraru (conflict) between the biological parents. I was also concerned that in the midst of that kōrero, the mana, mauri, and tapu of the children could be compromised if they were drawn into the adult conflict. It was better that they weren't part of that adult process.

Later during the kōrero, Tere used the word 'demonic'. I responded to this by saying that sometimes we are influenced by Christianity to believe that things we can't explain are demonic; however, I was sure that this situation was different. It was clear to me that this was a wake-up call for the whānau. I heard the kuia saying that if they would not look after this young lass, then she was going to 'take her'. This wake-up call was to tell the parents to reconcile their differences for the benefit of the children. Interestingly, the old lady took on two different forms during the course of our hui. At the beginning when I saw the old wahine (woman) she had longish grey hair and thin features. At the end of the interview, when Moana re-entered the room, I saw the same lady but this time she appeared younger and happier. At that moment my experience was that she seemed separate, slightly to the side of Moana, as if she had stepped back at that point, whereas at the beginning she appeared to be located within Moana, as if she was part of her. It was after the session when I next had an opportunity to speak to Allister that I came to understand that the old woman I heard and saw was actually Tere's great-great-grandmother.

During the session Tere kept referring to John, Moana's biological father, as 'he' and 'him'. I asked her to use his name, John, because he had a name and if they wanted to resolve whatever was happening to their daughter, then she could start that process right there. She took it upon herself with heaps of courage to speak directly to John for the first time and then asked for forgiveness for hurting him. She spoke about their daughters and how beautiful they were. So something really good came out of the reunion.

John replied when it came around to him. He acknowledged her in their own language. He talked about forgiveness. Acknowledging her in the Cook Islands Māori language was significant because this provided a korowai (cloak of protection) to the situation. It brought cultural and spiritual safety and in doing so, John was also acknowledging Tere's mana and the mana of her ancestors. He apologised to Tere's husband. Later, after I left, I was told that they spent another two hours together making up for the time that they had not been communicating. This suggested to me that an important reconciliation had begun.

Towards the end of the session I knew we needed to find a way to complete the process for that moment. From my point of view, in te ao Māori we would usually whakanoa a tapu process such as this with a hongi (pressing noses in greeting) and kai (sharing of food). This is about making a sacred process safe for ordinary interactions again. But for this setting, I suggested that the participants might choose to shake hands or embrace one another if they felt comfortable to do so as a way to whakanoa the reconciliation for the moment.

After this the children were asked to come back in. I was asked if we should karakia for Moana and I said no because she appeared to be different. I noticed that the taumaha, or heaviness, had been lifted off her. And so I declined and left it to the family, because with the reconciliation came the restoration of their mana, and it was well within their whānau to be able to resolve the situation. The minute that they had begun the reconciliation process there had been a spiritual shift.

Tere

Early in the meeting with Wiremu I needed to test him to find out if he really did have the spiritual awareness to help Moana and our family. I felt vulnerable and I needed to protect my family in case he wasn't the right person. When I asked him, 'What gender?' I was shocked when he replied, 'How did you get on with your grandmother?' How did he know about my great-great-grandmother? It was like having some layers peeled off. As well as feeling shocked, I felt more at ease and connected to him because he had that knowledge. I sensed he was strong enough to help us, that he wasn't going to take any crap!

Later, when Wiremu suggested that I start calling John by his name, it was like 'Ouch!' Someone had said something so truthful to me that I couldn't ignore it. I couldn't challenge it because he was so gentle about it but at the same time firm and sincere. By this time in our meeting I trusted him a lot because of the other things he knew. The trust between me and Wiremu had been built up over this short time as he knocked my walls down.

I found it very hard to turn to John and speak directly to him. Wiremu's presence there really helped me. He believed in me. What was in his eyes gave me courage. I was able to draw on the inner strength and spiritual strength that came out of him. I told myself, 'It has to happen now.'

The session that day helped with some kind of closure for what our family was going through. Having everyone there in the same room, having a child psychiatrist, a cultural therapist, a whole fruit salad there! It really helped that we could talk about it in front of a doctor and in front of a cultural person, knowing that what we were going through was okay. That was very compelling. Wiremu was able to put into words some things that I couldn't really understand in a way that helped me understand them. It was more powerful because he understood that spiritual stuff and the culture. Even though he was a New Zealand Māori he understood it. For example, he helped me see that the whole demonic thing was really a cultural thing. I was taken aback by that. It made me think again and helped me acknowledge and embrace a cultural view alongside my religious beliefs. It really made sense.

He also picked up that day that the stuff that Moana was going through was a lot of unresolved stuff between us as parents that had gone on to our child. I'd never spoken to him before, but he was explaining the story of what our family had been going through in a way that made sense. His explanation was like a familiar territory to me. I had my own experience of Moana's situation and I also knew about the things I experienced as I grew up.

As for Moana, the improvement in her state of mind after our session with Wiremu was dramatic. That same day it was like a whole weight had been peeled off her. She looked more peaceful than I had seen her for at least six months. She was much less anxious at night and sleeping much better. No more nightmares or worries. She began to bloom like a flower again. There were no more episodes of her becoming enraged—she was back to her normal caring, loving self again. She was able to communicate and talk about her feelings again like she had before all this happened.

If you were to ask me what of Wiremu's gifts led to the healing for our family, I would say it was all of his gifts. It was the package deal. His ability to see the spiritual side interacted with his healing understanding; that is, his knowing about what had to take place for healing to happen for our family. He was able to connect with all of us in a profound way and very quickly gain our trust. He was able to challenge us in a loving way. Most importantly for me, he acknowledged the relationship between all of us and God, our higher power. He said that he could do nothing without that and that anything good that came from our time together was not from him but came about through that authority. Without that nothing would happen. This acknowledgement was one reason I felt confident to trust him.

Some months after this meeting, Allister showed me a video of Wiremu speaking about what he had seen during the meeting that day. As well as the old woman, my great-great-grandmother whom he had mentioned that day, he described two men whom he hadn't talked about at that time. When I saw the video and heard his description, I wasn't sure who the men might be. But when I talked to my mother about it, she said that the descriptions fitted my grandfather and great-grandfather exactly. My grandfather, who died before my mother was born, was known for being clean-cut and large, and he often wore khaki shorts and a yellow singlet. Moana was named after him.

Allister

Just as I had been taken aback by George's rapid recovery after his single session with Wiremu in Chapter 4, I was not at all prepared for the transformation in Moana after Wiremu's only meeting with the family. Tere's description of the healing effect on her daughter and all the family was unequivocal, despite the differences between New Zealand Māori and Cook Islands culture and worldviews.

How can we account for this? Superficially, the methods Wiremu used to address this problem may resemble some family therapy approaches. However, it is evident from Wiremu's description that the basis for his decision to address the relational problem between Moana's parents was grounded in his spiritual discernment of her predicament. His method of assessment included perceptions not only of the appearance, intentions, and communications from family members in the therapy room, but also of deceased ancestors whom he perceived as present in the room.

A culturally appropriate way for a Cook Islands family to address a cultural problem might be to seek advice from a senior cultural authority from their own community. Although Wiremu made it clear that he could not profess to grasp the nuances of Cook Islands culture, language, meaning, and experience, there are some parallels in worldviews between New Zealand Māori and Cook Islands traditions, including understandings about concepts such as tapu (sacred or forbidden people, places, or processes) and mana (spiritual authority) (Baddeley, 1985), which are widely shared among cultures in the Pacific region. Maki tūpāpaku is an expression in the Cook Islands Māori language that refers to a kind of 'spirit illness' in which the sufferer may be affected by strange behaviour and severe emotional distress (Baddeley, 1985). From a Cook Islands perspective, such afflictions are often viewed as resulting from a breakdown in social or family relationships. Ta'unga (Cook Islands traditional healers) have been described as commonly spending a great deal of time consulting with the affected family, facilitating the resolution of any unresolved matters such as grievances or conflict that are viewed as being at the heart of the problem (Baddeley, 1985). In this way the 'sick person' in this context is helped by a process of family healing rather than being treated in isolation.

These Cook Islands perspectives have similarities to Wiremu's New Zealand Māori worldview. Such links, along with his spiritual insights and understanding of the family's predicament, his articulation of the identified cause of this, his ability to connect strongly and empathically with both estranged parents, and to use his own mana and mauri to encourage a change during the session, seemed to be key factors in the healing experienced by this family.

The methods that Wiremu used are consistent with descriptions of the practice of tohunga from several sources (Durie, 2009; Mark & Lyons, 2010; Moon, 2003; Parsons, 1985). It is commonly accepted in New Zealand Māori communities that certain individuals have the ability to perceive communications from deceased ancestors, and it is expected that tohunga may use such abilities as part of their therapeutic assessment. Similarly, descriptions of traditional healing work in the Cook Islands indicate that ta'unga are also commonly accepted as having such abilities (Baddeley, 1985).

In both Cook Islands and New Zealand Māori traditions, frequently identified causes of spiritual distress include relational breaches or conflicts, and the appropriate remedy may therefore include ways of healing such breaches. A similar philosophy can be found among other cultures indigenous to the Pacific region, whereby breaches may be understood to be intergenerational and may involve both the living and the dead (Tamasese et al., 2005). In these cases and consistent with these philosophies, spiritual reparation, relational reconciliation, and seeking forgiveness and atonement are often viewed as appropriate ways of alleviating distress. Ultimately the focus is to address breaches, release burdens, and restore and rebalance relational harmony in ways that are positive for all.

Notes

1. Moana's story has previously been published in a family therapy journal (NiaNia et al., 2013).
2. Maki tūpāpaku is a Cook Islands Māori expression that refers to a form of spirit possession.
3. The Cook Islands comprise 15 islands spread across more than two million square kilometres in the middle of the South Pacific Ocean. This nation is self-governing and has a long-standing close political relationship with New Zealand. The capital, Avarua, is situated on the island of Rarotonga. The Cook Islands Māori language is also known as te reo Ipukarea, or Rarotongan, and includes a number of dialects.

References

Baddeley, J. (1985). 'Traditional healing practices of Rarotonga, Cook Islands'. Chapter 7 in Parsons, C.D.F. (ed.), *Healing practices in the South Pacific*, pp. 129–43. University of Hawai'i Press, Honolulu.

Bush, A., Chapman, F., Drummond, M. & Fagaloa, T. (2009) 'Development of a child, adolescent and family mental health service for Pacific young people in Aotearoa/New Zealand'. *Pacific Health Dialog* 15: 138–46.

Durie, M. (2009). 'Maori knowledge and medical science: The interface between psychiatry and traditional healing in New Zealand'. Chapter 19 in Incayawar, M., Wintrob, R. & Bouchard, L. (eds), *Psychiatrists and traditional healers: Unwitting partners in global mental health*, pp. 237–49. John Wiley & Sons, Chichester.

Mark, G.T. & Lyons, A.C. (2010) 'Maori healers' views on wellbeing: The importance of mind, body, spirit, family and land'. *Social Science & Medicine* 70: 1756–64.

Moon, P. (2003) *Tohunga Hohepa Kereopa*. David Ling Publishing, Auckland.

NiaNia, W., Tere, Bush A. & Epston, D. (2013) '"I will not leave my baby behind": A Cook Island Māori family's experience of New Zealand Māori traditional healing'. *Australian and New Zealand Journal of Family Therapy* 34: 3–17.

Parsons, C.D.F. (1985) 'Notes on Maori sickness knowledge and healing practices'. Chapter 11 in Parsons, C.D.F. (ed.), *Healing practices in the South Pacific*, pp. 213–34. University of Hawai'i Press, Honolulu.

Tamasese, K., Peteru, C., Waldegrave, C. & Bush, A. (2005) 'Ole Taeao Afua, the new morning: A qualitative investigation into Samoan perspectives on mental health and culturally appropriate services'. *Australian and New Zealand Journal of Psychiatry* 39: 300–09.

Waldegrave, C., Tamasese, K., Tuhaka, F. & Campbell, W. (2003) *Just Therapy- a journey: A collection of papers from the Just Therapy Team, New Zealand*. Dulwich Centre Publications, Adelaide.

7

INTO THE WORLD OF LIGHT

Anyone who has worked with troubled teenagers will know that sometimes finding a resolution is not simple or quick. There may be many ups and downs during a young person's involvement with mental health services. In previous chapters we have seen situations in which a single session with Wiremu led to immediate relief. In this chapter we describe Wiremu's healing work over an extended period with a teenager called Tangi. In particular, Tangi's story illustrates a holistic approach in which Wiremu as the Māori healer works alongside Allister as Tangi's psychiatrist and other team members, including hospital psychiatry staff, in a collaboration that addresses Tangi's spiritual, psychological, physical, and family well-being.

The narrative begins by introducing us to Tangi and what led to the distress she was experiencing at the time of her initial meetings with her therapist and psychiatrist. It recounts her progress in therapy over the first year and our awareness that she is a spiritually attuned young person.

The story then focuses on Wiremu's involvement. The second part of the chapter documents in detail the first three sessions that Tangi had with Wiremu. During the first, he provides a cultural context for Tangi's puzzling spiritual experiences, explains Māori constructs that help her navigate this unfamiliar terrain, and encourages her to take Māori stories and symbols inherent in her artwork and move them in a healing direction.

Shortly after, things take a turn for the worse for Tangi. In the second session, Wiremu identifies the spiritual problem that he perceives is impinging on her. The narrative tells of Tangi's decision, Wiremu's intervention at the end of the third session, and Tangi's period of well-being over the next six months.

It is then that she begins to experience new voices and visions that become very distressing for her until they reach such an intensity that she agrees to be admitted to an adolescent psychiatry hospital unit.

In the third part of the chapter, we see how Wiremu continues to work alongside Tangi and collaborate closely with the hospital team. From a psychiatry point of view, it appears that Tangi is suffering from a severe psychotic illness. However, Wiremu describes the spiritual perceptions that convince him Tangi is suffering primarily from a spiritual problem and that the path to well-being requires a spiritual solution, alongside medication and other hospital treatment that Tangi is receiving. This unusual collaborative approach, involving hospital psychiatry clinicians, community clinicians, and Wiremu as her Māori healer, allows Tangi's distress to be safely contained, and over time she begins to recover. The hospital team include Wiremu's assessment findings in their understanding of Tangi's predicament, and together an integrated approach incorporating medical, psychological, and spiritual aspects contribute to her steady recovery.

The chapter then turns to Wiremu's account of Tangi's spiritual problem and her renewed well-being. Next Tangi offers her own perspective on her experiences, her healing relationship with Wiremu, and her new journey in a vocation that she is passionate about. In particular Tangi articulates the enabling change she experiences in Wiremu's approach as he invites her to step into a more authoritative stance in relation to her spiritual world. The chapter ends with reference to the mental health literature to shed light on Tangi's story in relation to recent research on the experience of people who hear voices.

Allister

Introducing Tangi

Tangi was 16 years old when she was first seen at our Māori Child, Adolescent and Family Service (Māori CAFS), 18 months before her initial meeting with Wiremu. Her mother had referred her because she had become concerned about her daughter's well-being over the previous six months. Tangi had become tearful and unhappy and at other times unpredictably angry. She was withdrawing from her friends and spending more and more time alone in her room, and she was fighting with her younger sisters and brother every day. At her first appointment with Jade, her Māori CAFS social worker, she spoke openly for the first time of her deepening unhappiness over the previous three years.

Tangi was the oldest grandchild of her Koro (grandfather) and Nan, who both came from the same traditional iwi area on the East Coast of New Zealand. She had always known that she was the apple of her Koro's eye, even though he wasn't one to show his affection too openly. As with many first-born Māori grandchildren, her Koro and Nan had asserted their caregiving role in her infancy, which inadvertently resulted in her mother feeling uncertain about her own place as Tangi's mother.

Tangi considered that Koro had been like a father to her, and she had been in his company almost every day. She adored Koro and Nan's two Jack Russell terriers, Tama and Poppy. These relationships had cushioned her when she was five years old from the loss that followed her parents' separation and her father's subsequent emigration to Australia. Even though she didn't think he'd been the perfect dad, she really missed him. After he left, she would see him sometimes in holidays when he would come to visit or when she stayed with him and his new family. She excelled in sport and regretted that he wasn't on the sidelines of the hockey field every Saturday to watch her play, like other fathers.

At the age of 13, Tangi was overjoyed when her father raised the prospect of her coming to live with him and his new family in Australia near a sports academy at a local college. However, within months of moving in with him, her high hopes turned to disillusionment when she realised that the college didn't have the right programme for her sporting ambitions. Before long she was skipping classes, and tension mounted in her relationship with her father. She missed Tama and Poppy and felt more and more lonely, isolated, and depressed. After a very contentious argument with her father, she was sent back to her whānau in Aotearoa.

On her return, Tangi was relieved to be reunited with her whānau and animal companions, and for a while all was well. She caught up with old friends. However, before long she was horrified to discover that she was pregnant after a brief relationship. Tangi described this as her 'lowest point'. She knew she didn't want to proceed with the pregnancy; as she recalled it: 'It felt like I had something alien inside me.' At the same time, though, she didn't want to hurt the baby. When the subject of a termination was raised, Tangi felt caught in an impossible dilemma. Pressure mounted for her to make a decision. Her whānau, who considered her too young to proceed with the pregnancy, encouraged her to go ahead with the procedure, and finally she reluctantly agreed.

Tangi's first meeting with Jade, her Māori CAFS social worker, was a year later. As she talked, all the troubles of those 12 difficult months spilled out. She felt so isolated from close whānau members, even though they seemed to want to be there for her. She avoided her old friends and came to believe they were turning against her. She even came to the sad conclusion that her beloved animal companions, Tama and Poppy, were intentionally shunning her. She withdrew from sporting activities that had always been her passion. She felt so desperate and lost that at one point she tried to end her life, and occasionally she secretly cut herself with a razor at home. At other times she would smoke marijuana that she obtained from someone at school. These activities provided temporary relief, but couldn't distract her for long from the self-condemnation that was consuming her. She was tormented by nightmares about death, about the termination, and about people close to her perishing. The nightmares were accompanied by dreams of people being assaulted, reminding her of family violence she had witnessed.

Around this time Tangi had returned to school after the summer holidays. Then, seemingly out of the blue, she experienced her first panic attacks. The first occurred in class when, without warning, they were invited to watch a movie about childbirth. During the screening, she felt overcome with guilt. Her palms became hot and sweaty, her heart was pounding, and she was growing short of breath. Overwhelmed by panic and fearing for her life, she fled the classroom. After some time, Tangi managed to calm herself down and return to class. But the panic returned within a few days and then became a regular occurrence. These episodes compounded her private sense of powerlessness in her life and fed the hopelessness and worthlessness she had been trying to resist. Thoughts of ending her life returned to plague her.

As Tangi allowed herself to trust Jade over their first few sessions, she revealed more about her private suffering. Jade realised Tangi had enough symptoms to justify a diagnosis of depression. She helped Tangi practise slowing her breathing to manage her feelings of panic, and together they met up with the school guidance counsellor to plan how she could manage episodes at school. Tangi was reluctant to involve her family, but Jade persuaded her they should talk to her mother to help support her with the safety plan that they were working on, so her mother could assist her in her most desperate moments. After meeting Jade, Tangi's feeling of desperation seemed to ease somewhat, and she appreciated having someone to confide in. To her relief, she regained a sense of control when panicky feelings came up.

Jade and I both met with Tangi several weeks later. At this time, Tangi talked about feeling different from her whānau and peers. She described frequent experiences that she believed were spiritual in nature, which she hadn't shared with whānau because she was afraid they would say she was 'mental'. She spoke of a 'white thing' at her Koro's house that she had come to believe was a deceased family member. She described it as a friendly presence, which she could locate in space. She talked of seeing a 'brown thing' also at her Koro's place, which again she had identified—this time as a deceased uncle who had died very young. Again she was untroubled by this 'thing'. In contrast to these benign experiences, after her termination she had noticed a 'black thing' hanging around her. Tangi considered this some kind of curse related to the termination. She'd wondered if it was the spirit of her baby watching her. At some moments she would hear a rubbing sound when it was there or a sound like banging on the wall. She occasionally heard whispers but no understandable speech. The 'black thing' seemed to have some kind of malevolent intent, and at one point she was sure that her dog Tama had growled at it.

Tangi talked about other experiences that she believed were spiritual. She spoke of a dream in which a friend prepared to hang herself; the same day she visited this friend, noticed the rope, and realised her friend was close to suicide. Because of this premonition, Tangi was able to intervene and seek help for her friend.

When we discussed her depressed mood and other symptoms, I also came to the conclusion that a diagnosis of depression was justified. Despite unusual perceptual experiences that she considered spiritual, Tangi had no other symptoms indicating a psychotic illness, such as delusions or disorganised thinking or behaviour. Her panic attacks persisted at school, but she was becoming more adept at calming herself and managing these. Her bad dreams suggested a traumatic origin, especially the ones in which she would reexperience violence she had witnessed in her early years. Although we discussed possible medication to address her depression, Tangi was positive about meeting with Jade and believed these therapy sessions were already helping her.

A while later Tangi experienced a setback after a row at home with her siblings. She felt that her mother, Koro, and Nan had all sided with her siblings, and the old feelings of isolation returned. Her mood plummeted again and she had strong urges to end her life, with thoughts of hanging herself. She disclosed to Jade for the first time that she had been sniffing petrol in the garage to block out her feelings of despair and desolation and had been cutting herself again. The panic episodes also flared up at school.

As a result of these problems, Tangi decided she would like to try the antidepressant medication. This treatment, combined with Tangi's therapy with Jade, seemed to contribute to a steady improvement in her mood. Her panic episodes settled down. At this time, Jade persuaded Tangi to allow her Nan and Koro to attend some sessions, which led to a positive shift in her Koro and Nan's way of relating to her, especially when she was feeling low or moody. In their individual sessions, Jade introduced mindfulness exercises to assist Tangi manage strong negative feelings that overwhelmed her when she resorted to cutting herself and sniffing petrol.[1] Because of Tangi's strong interest in art, they embarked on a Māori therapeutic approach known as Te Tuakiri o te Ora. This is a structured, art-based therapy that is centred on exploration of nine significant Māori kupu, or concepts, which the young person is encouraged to consider in light of narratives from their own life. This therapy focuses on a gentle exploration of the young person's sense of identity, including cultural identity, and there is space for their reflection on a broad range of themes such as mana, mauri, tapu, spirituality, and whatumanawa (deep-seated emotions). Matters of grief and loss often surface during the course of this work.

Over the course of her therapy with Jade, Tangi often returned to the pain of her guilt and shame about the termination. The more she returned to it, the more the intense, painful memories eased. As she explored her spiritual experiences, she learnt to view these as a vital part of who she was. The themes in her Tuakiri artwork frequently touched on relationships with her mother and father and other family members. She seemed to become stronger in her sense of self and appeared less troubled at times of conflict if family members used insults such as calling her 'mental'. The moments when she felt a strong urge to cut herself or sniff petrol became few and far between.

Prior to the first session with Wiremu, Jade had begun to discuss with Tangi the end of the therapy and a date for discharge from our service. Meanwhile

Jade was preparing to take a year's maternity leave. However, not long after, Jade became concerned about a number of matters that Tangi was describing. Although her mood was 'okay' most days, she talked about seeing 'the black thing' around again and feeling troubled by this. After a verbal fight with her mother, she cut herself on the arm—and she repeated this several times over several days. When an opportunity to consult with Wiremu came up, Tangi was keen to meet him.

Wiremu's First Session with Tangi

Tangi arrived early for the appointment with Wiremu. She was dressed in jeans and a T-shirt and carrying her schoolbag and two poi, because she had kapa haka (Māori performing group) training later in the day. When Wiremu arrived, he joined Jade, Tangi, and me, as well as a trainee doctor who Tangi had agreed could sit in. When we were all seated Wiremu asked me to say a karakia to start the session. After this it was time for a mihi whakatau (round of introductions). Wiremu then requested that someone speak about how things had been for Tangi during the time she had been at Te Whare Mārie. Tangi asked if either Jade or I could do that on her behalf. Jade summarised Tangi's concerns, all the while checking with Tangi for confirmation, which she did by nodding.

Tangi then talked about a trip to her home marae the previous summer and how she found it scary because of things she felt there. Wiremu reassured her that it was common to feel scared around marae, especially if you weren't brought up there. He explained that it was her Koro's role to help her with that. He then asked her about her whānau names and connections on the East Coast, and when she responded he acknowledged that he was familiar with the whānau and her home marae.

We join the session as Wiremu steers the conversation towards an exploration of one of the spiritual experiences that he has been told is troubling for Tangi.

Wiremu: This black thing. Does it scare you?

Tangi: Not any more. It used to. But it's not here anymore. It's moved on. That's how I think about it. It went into the light. There are still other spirits lingering around. I don't really like to talk about it because people at school find it weird.

Wiremu: It's not at all.

Tangi: They don't get it. (Wiremu laughs). I always get kicked out if I talk about it. I just keep it to myself. I just think about it, write about it, that's about it. When I go into hospitals, I just feel scary stuff. So I don't go into hospitals. I don't go into graveyards. I don't like to go to marae and I don't like to go to funerals.

Wiremu: You don't like going to funerals?

Tangi: Nah, not because of the sadness, but because of the spiritual side.

Wiremu: I don't like going to funerals either, but I guess I'll have to go to my own! (laughter)

At this point Wiremu asks Jade how, in her opinion, Tangi is progressing. Jade talks about a number of areas in Tangi's life where she has noticed Tangi making steps forward in reclaiming her life. Then, almost as an aside, she comments on what she perceives as some loneliness in Tangi's life.

Jade: It's felt a bit like your whānau just don't get you sometimes, eh? Except for the dogs, Tama and Poppy, they get you.
Tangi: Even Tama has been distancing himself from me recently.
Wiremu: Dogs are good friends alright. It's a bit hard if you haven't got anyone to talk to about this stuff.
Jade: You were really worried about what Koro would think about you coming here and seeing us and what it would mean for him.

Wiremu then asks about the involvement of Tangi's whānau in the therapy so far and comments that it would be very important for her Koro and Nan to have an understanding of what has been happening for her. He learns that her Koro had a strong paternal role in her upbringing.

Wiremu: Does he kōrero Māori?
Tangi: He used to but when I went to school and learnt English I kind of lost it. So he doesn't kōrero Māori to me anymore. Just a little bit. But he's like the old, old style . . .
Wiremu: Those Ngāti Porou fellas are like that.
Tangi: He gets hōhā (annoyed) if I don't get it right.
Wiremu: I think some of them up the coast are still riding their horses into the pub!
Tangi: They are!
Wiremu: Real staunch!
Tangi: Mum says they are a proud family. That's why Mum wants us to do something great. That's what she always tried to get us to do.
Wiremu: Well, if Jade says your Tuakiri art therapy was awesome, I believe it. And art must be a place for greatness. Actually I wouldn't have minded meeting your Koro. I like those staunch kind of Ngāti Porou fellas! I've met a few while I've been down here who've lost touch with their tūrangawaewae, their home. So they get grouchy.
Tangi: Yeah! Real grouchy!
Wiremu: 'Remember back in the day?' That's their kōrero.
Tangi: It's cool going back up there. We've got our little farm and house that my Koro's sister looks after. We have Māori bread and tea all the time.
Wiremu: Who does the baking?

Tangi: Nan, not me. I have to do the work with Koro. I like doing the farm work.

Wiremu: So, have you told these fellas how you can be helped or how they can help you?

Wiremu, having encouraged Tangi to talk about her doubts and fears about visiting her home marae, then offers some details of cultural context that help explain her Koro's responses. Wiremu's comments seem to make sense to her, and she then talks warmly about her experience of being up on the family farm on the East Coast where her whānau come from. As she tunes in to this positive experience of herself and her places of belonging, Wiremu invites her to offer the team some direction on what kind of help she would like. Wiremu frequently works to enhance the mana of people he is working with, and here he creates an opportunity for Tangi to experience being in charge of key decisions about the direction of the therapeutic work.

Later in the session Wiremu decides to address the question of Tangi's termination and what this means to her. He has heard from Jade that she blamed herself for this and, although her previous intense feelings of guilt have lessened, she still feels sensitive about this matter.

Wiremu: You know, given that you had the termination, Tangi, one of the things that I wanted to say was that the way I see it, things die in order for other things to grow. The death of something is not the end. It means something that's good is going to come out of that. Even if your Koro, or someone who you treasure or love passes away, you may feel that loss deeply. However, even for a loss as painful as that, something good is going to come out of that.

I'll talk about myself. If I lost someone very dear to me, I would strive to ensure that I'm going to become better at some of the things I intend to put my hand to. In your case, I'm not sure if that's the sport or the kapahaka or the art. I can see that you're good at kapahaka, just from your stance, your body language. I know that something good is going to come out of the experience you've had. Not just average, I mean really good. So, I'll probably come back in a couple of years' time and get your autograph!

At this point Wiremu moves on to address the question of Tangi and her spiritual awareness. He explains that this kind of gift is common in the traditional area where her whānau come from. He explains that negative spiritual influences can often latch on to a young person with the most potential.

Wiremu: They would like to keep you as an underachiever in order to control or manipulate. I'm hearing that your whānau may be pinning some hopes on you achieving something great. So in order to damage a whole family, they will pick on the one who is able to achieve something for the whānau. If you kōrero to whānau who have been affected like this, they might have pinned their hopes on one of their whānau to achieve something to bring status to the whānau, and they find that somewhere along the line, drugs or sniffing or boozing has actually stunted that.

I think I talk too much!

Tangi: (in a singsong tone) You got it!

Wiremu: That I talk too much?

Tangi: No! (laughter all round) Someone who actually understands.

A few moments later there is a natural pause in the conversation, and I take this opportunity to invite Wiremu to comment on a matter that I have been wondering about.

Allister: I'm interested in the connection between depression and the black thing. How are these things connected? Is the depression sometimes caused by the black thing? What would you say, Wiremu?

Wiremu: In te ao Māori, first there was Hineahuone. She was known as the earth maiden. And she had a daughter called Hinetītama, who became the dawn maiden.

Tangi: I love stories!

Wiremu: Now somewhere along the line Hinetītama was incestuously interfered with. When she found out that it was actually her dad who was her lover, Hinetītama became depressed because she was traumatised by that fact. I believe this is where the word hinengaro came from. It comes from that lost and depressed state that Hinetītama experienced. Then, because there was no way back for her, she progressed on to become Hinenuitepō. There was no one there to help her come out of that state of hinengaro. Hinenuitepō lives in the very darkest depths, the blackness. So I firmly believe that the stage to intervene is now. Otherwise, that 'thing' (I call them 'things' or 'gremlins') will pull you to that depth.

These 'things' have been around for ages and ages. They know what makes us tick. They know what sets us off. They know how to push our buttons, and they also know when you have the potential to help others. Because of that they create dissension, they become disruptive. Your black thing is part of that. I don't know whether this is making sense.

Tangi: It is!

Jade: They pick on the strongest ones, then?

Wiremu: Yes, they try to bring them down any way they can.

Allister: Can you sense any kind of black thing around Tangi at the moment?

Wiremu: No. Not right here. Not right now. They tend to hide. That's why I just like sitting in the quietness. And again, I believe the eyes are the gateway to the soul. And so, if I look at someone, usually I can pick up what's behind their eyes. Actually there's nothing there at the moment. I'm not saying you haven't got any brains or anything! (laughter) I'm saying the black thing isn't there.

Tangi: It's not there, because he knows that there's . . .

Wiremu: (earnestly interrupting) Its hold is not so great, but it's lurking. Let me say it's lurking. That's why I'm keen to karakia for you before we close up, because I really love giving them a good going-over.

Jade: (to Tangi) There was a brown thing and a white thing that you spoke of when we first met. They seemed a bit more positive.

Tangi: The brown one was my Uncle Harold, who died two days after he was born. And the white one was my Nana Pat. She died of breast cancer. I didn't know what the brown thing was until he told me. Then I asked Mum more about him and found out who he was.

But I want to say something else. That story that you told about Hinenuitepō. My art has been based around Hinenuitepō these last two months! And now I've just made a connection about Hinenuitepō and the black thing and my art, and how it connects together in my life. And how Hinenuitepō has just come in and I didn't really realise it.

Jade: Far out!

(This is the first that Jade and I have heard of this theme in Tangi's artwork.)

Wiremu: Gee, I'd love to see your art! You know how your art has been about Hinenuitepō. I wonder if you would be able to step back and start to bring her out of the darkness. One way could be to bring her back to Hinengaro. Hinengaro is often taken as referring to the psychological or emotional or mental side of who we are, and we often use expressions like 'all in the hinengaro', which is referring to mental well-being.

Allister: Tangi, I know you have heard that term 'mental' being used in a bad way. Wiremu, are you meaning the mind when you talk about mental well-being?

Wiremu: Yes. That side of us. We have the mind. We have the body. We have the whānau. And we have the . . . what's the other one?

Allister: Wairua.

Wiremu: Whoa! How could I miss that? (laughter all round) But yeah, we have these four sides. That's who we are as people. However, hinengaro is the least understood of the four. If we think of hine as being the female gender—which comes from Hineahuone and Hinetītama—and ngaro as being 'lost', or things obscured or hidden. You have a chance to bring her back, from Hinenuitepō to Hinengaro and then to Hinetītama, which is the dawn maiden. I hope I get a chance to see your art sometime!

Later in the interview Wiremu explained mauri, tapu, and mana:

Wiremu: Mauri is often described as the 'life force'. It is about being whole, it is about your whakapapa, it is what keeps you moving and keeps you motivated. The kupu mauri is made up of two parts, 'ma' and 'uri'. 'Uri' refers to kin or kinship relationships. 'Ma' as in mā tēnā, means 'by that'. So ma-uri taken together can be translated as 'by that relationship'. So my relationship with my whānau, or my children or my other relationships, constitutes my life force. But mauri goes a lot higher than that. If I turn heavenward, I would say that it is about my relationship with God, or God's relationship with me.

The next word for us to look at is tapu. If we split the word tapu into two parts, ta and pu, then 'ta' is from 'tā' which means 'to fashion' or 'to carve'. We talk about 'tā moko' [Māori tattooing]. Widows back in the old days, if their husband died, they'd get a tattoo carved on their chin. They would have what is called a moko kauae. This tā moko signified that this was a person of stature or status and where they came from. When I think of your youth-group learnings about the Bible, then I think of a quote from the book of Isaiah that says that the creator has carved us into the palm of his hand. This symbolism helps me understand the link between the word 'tā' and my creator or source. The second part, 'pu' is from 'pū' as contained in the waiata: 'Ko te pū, te more, te weu'—that's the beginning of the root systems. 'Pu' can be taken to refer to the beginning or the origin. Again, if I were to relate this to biblical themes, then there is the metaphor of Christ as the vine. He's the vine that brings life. So 'pu' could be taken to refer to the origin or the source. So here we have 'ta' and 'pu'. Tapu is often translated as sacred. It actually goes way beyond that. Going back to that biblical reference, if he is the source, then it says, 'I the source have graven you into the palm of my hand.' That is a very close and personal relationship with the creator. And this idea takes it way beyond just being 'sacred'.

Then we get to this word mana. Mana is often viewed as being an authority, power, or prestige. Because of our relationship with the creator and the sacredness of that, God has given me and you the authority to have dominion over everything that walks, creeps, crawls, flies, and swims. It gives you the authority to be in charge of any situation you are in. That mana gives you the authority to be spiritually in charge of your space. You can be selective about what you see and hear, and when you get to where you are going with your youth group then you'll know that that black thing will have no hold over you. You can tell it where to go. And you can claim back that which you have lost. If anything has been taken away through grief, you can claim that back. You can say, 'I don't have to accept this because I'm in charge here.' Does that make sense?

Tangi: Yes, everything you've said I understand and it does make sense.

After this Wiremu asks the trainee doctor if she has any comments. She says that she has noticed that during the session it seems a special connection has developed between Tangi and Wiremu. Tangi responds to this comment:

Tangi: I wasn't sure at first, but now I can feel that connection. And I know when you are seeing into me. I know when you are doing that. And I know when you are trying to find something in me. It's really cool! Because no one ever does that to me. So thanks!

Here Tangi describes something unique in her experience of the session with Wiremu. She appears to be describing her awareness of him 'seeing into' her, which she then reports as a positive experience.

Wiremu finishes the session by bringing the conversation back to Tangi and her art and hockey. He says that he is not sure if they will meet again, but he will be asking Jade how she is getting on:

Wiremu: I still want to keep up with you and your art and your hockey. I'll be asking Jade now and again: 'How's that Tangi? When can I get her autograph?'

Shortly after the Session

Within a brief space of time, Jade became alarmed about a number of changes in Tangi. Whereas previously Tangi had been open and easy to relate to, almost overnight she seemed mistrustful. She had always made easy eye contact with Jade, but now her head was down and she wouldn't look Jade in the eyes. Tangi appeared troubled by something but very reluctant to talk about it. Finally she revealed that she had been hearing a voice telling her to kill her family members and not to talk to Jade. Jade arranged an urgent appointment for the three of us to meet up.

I, too, was puzzled and concerned about the dramatic change in Tangi's demeanour. She sat with her head down and wouldn't look at me. The spontaneous humour and sparkle that I'd seen in Tangi of late were nowhere to be seen. Whereas previously she had eloquently described her experiences and emotions, now she was unable to put words to what was going on for her. I wondered if she was upset about Jade's imminent departure on maternity leave. When I gently approached this topic, she had no comment. Finally she spoke about the voice. Immediately after this she put her hands over her ears and curled up almost in a foetal posture. Eventually she explained that the voice was yelling at her and demanding that she stop talking to us and 'shut up!' She described the voice as a male. It sounded to her just as real as our voices. Its origin seemed to be somewhere in the room around her.

She told us the voice was very familiar to her. It had been her frequent companion for many years. She remembered its presence back in primary school, assuring her when she was lonely it was her only true friend. It seemed jealous of her friendships with others and would encourage her not to trust those around her. Sometimes it would tell her to do cruel things. Years before, she told us, this same voice had instructed her to drown a kitten and she had gone ahead with this demand and felt terrible afterwards. In moments when she felt enraged with her brothers and sisters, the voice would goad her into hurting them. At various times in her life, it had told her to kill members of her family. Sometimes, as a result, she had lashed out more violently, and once she had tried to stab her brother with a knife. After incidents like this, her whānau would call her 'mental', and this only served to increase her sense of isolation.

Tangi told us that the voice had been mysteriously absent at the time of her hui with Wiremu, but returned with a vengeance a few days later. On the day of our appointment she recalled that the voice was there beside her as she lay in bed after waking, carrying on its usual conversation, greeting her with 'Hi', and 'I hope you had a good sleep' and informing her, 'I'm coming with you to see Jade.' It instructed her to 'get up!' and during the appointment had been telling her, 'Don't look at either of them, they're going to kill you!'

Both Jade and I were very surprised to hear Tangi's account of the voice and its pervasive role in her life: she had not spoken about it over the previous 18 months. Tangi explained that she had kept silent about it because she was afraid that we would think she was 'mental' and, in fact, she had been afraid that was indeed the case. I felt alarmed about the voice's demands that she kill those with whom she was angry. Even in our interview it was apparent that the voice could exert a strong influence on her as she seemed to be subject to an intense internal struggle about whether to disclose its presence to us or not.

From my perspective as a psychiatrist, the most likely explanation for Tangi's voice was that it was an auditory hallucination, and a dangerous one at that, heralding possibly the manifestation of a serious psychotic illness. Although such a symptom could occur if a young person was abusing substances, Tangi said that if anything she had been using less marijuana in the previous few weeks. The dramatic and sudden nature of Tangi's disclosure in the lead-up to Jade's departure even led me to briefly consider that she might have fabricated it as a reason to maintain her involvement with our service. However, I soon dismissed that idea as she described in detail the voice's influence in her life over a long period. I was puzzled that these experiences had become so intense within two weeks of seeing Wiremu. Perhaps that timing made a spiritual cause less likely, but if it was psychosis, I was at a loss to explain the sudden increase in intensity of her symptoms.

At the end of the appointment I explained to Tangi that I could think of three possible explanations for the voice. One was that it was an auditory hallucination that was being caused by some kind of 'psychosis'. I explained to her that psychosis is a kind of illness in which the mind begins to perceive things that don't have a basis in reality outside the person's mind. Even severe depression could be a cause of this, but as her mood hadn't recently been depressed, this wasn't likely to be the cause in her case. A second explanation was that the voice was an auditory hallucination caused by a kind of dissociation, which is a way that the mind can protect itself when it has had to cope with some serious trauma. And the third possibility was that the voice could be caused by a wairua or mate Māori problem. My reason for seriously considering a wairua explanation in this situation was my experience of working with George two years before and the dramatic nature of the voice he experienced and its sudden resolution after Wiremu's intervention. Nevertheless, everything in my psychiatric training told me that this had to be considered a psychotic problem until proven otherwise.

Interestingly, Tangi's response to this explanation was that she didn't think this was a wairua problem because it didn't seem like any of her other wairua experiences. She was concerned that the voice must mean that she had schizophrenia. When I talked with her about schizophrenia and explained that she didn't have the other symptoms that would be required to make this diagnosis, such as delusions or disorganised thinking or behaviour, then she seemed to relax and became much more spontaneous.

It would be another three weeks before we could consult with Wiremu again. In the meantime we agreed on a plan to keep Tangi and her family safe. When I talked about possible antipsychotic medication treatment as a way of reducing and hopefully stopping a psychotic symptom like this voice, Tangi decided she wanted to go ahead with this. I explained the side effects and that the benefits may take a week or two to be noticeable and prescribed a low dose of risperidone once daily for her.

Tangi's mother joined us for the final part of the appointment and was very concerned when she was informed about the voice that Tangi was experiencing. However, she did say it helped explain some of Tangi's angry and violent behaviour at home. Her biggest concern was that Tangi would stop communicating with the family when she was at her most distressed. Consequently, we assisted Tangi and her mother to negotiate a way of communicating about her degree of safety in those moments and what her mother could do to support her if needed and when to contact the mental health service for extra assistance.

Both Jade and I had been considering offering Tangi crisis respite or even a hospital admission because of the voice's injunctions to kill others. However, by the end of the appointment, Tangi seemed suddenly more spontaneous in her involvement and said she had plans for the weekend. She declared that the voice had been telling her to do these things for many years and she felt that she could handle it until our next meeting. When Jade and I reiterated our doubts and concerns, Tangi said she would ignore the voices or listen to music to drown them out, as she had done many times before, and she endeavoured to persuade her mother that she would be safe at home. At this point her mother agreed, and Jade arranged for daily visits to review this safety plan with them both.

By two weeks later, Tangi reported that she was sleeping better and the voice had begun to fade. It now sounded like it was talking to her from behind a wall to her left side. It was less intense, but still definitely there. Tangi persisted in withdrawing to her bedroom, and her mother remained very worried, especially about what the voice meant in terms of a possible psychotic illness and whether Tangi would act on her thoughts to harm others in the family. Although the voice was still suggesting that she hurt others when she felt angry, she said she was finding it easy to resist these directions. I was reassured that she seemed more relaxed and trusting in our meeting and was able to look at me. She was no longer resorting to blocking her ears or turning away. As a result, we agreed to continue the same plan until we could meet with Wiremu.

Second Session with Wiremu

Tangi's second session with Wiremu is one month after the first. The night before, her mother has rung the crisis team for assistance as she is alarmed at Tangi's talk about wanting to kill members of her family.

Tangi's Nan brings her in for the session for the first time. She seems eager to meet Wiremu, and we invite her in with Tangi for the first part of the session. Wiremu asks if I can start our session with a karakia and then there is a mihi whakatau (round of introductions). Tangi's Nan and Wiremu spend some time talking about their family links from the East Coast, and then Nan speaks in detail about her concerns for Tangi over a long period and their close relationship with her.

After Tangi's Nan leaves the room, I explain to Tangi that we have heard about the phone call and arrange with her that Jade and I will see her after Wiremu's session to talk to her about keeping her and the family safe at home. Then I ask Tangi if she was okay with us bringing Wiremu up to date with recent developments. She agrees and asks that I do so.

I brief Wiremu, with Tangi's help, about the voice that Tangi has reported and what it has been saying. I talk about our dilemma about whether this voice is a psychotic symptom or whether it could possibly be a spiritual problem. I explain that Tangi has said that she doesn't think it is spiritual.

Wiremu then invites Tangi to talk about her experience of the voice.

Tangi: I don't know what I think. Sometimes I think it's the voice in my head that thinks for me. I told Mum, it's like another me. It's like two me's. And it just comes out stronger. He pushes me out. He comes and gets me to say all those words like I did last night.

Allister: Do you mean about killing people?

Tangi: Yeah. I'll be angry. It'll be him that will rark me up. Once there's nothing to do, I'll come back and it'll be normal me again. Mum asked about that. She was scared about if it was really me. Then when I am me, he's just in my head, telling me things, or sometimes it feels like he's right next to me.

Allister: Do you sometimes hear the voice outside of yourself?

Tangi: Yeah. It's about half and half. And it's changed since I've been taking that medication. Now it sounds like there is a wall here (indicating a wall to the left of her) that's blocking him out so that his voice sounds kind of muffled. Also, since then I've been seeing some things that are weird. Sometimes I'll see bright shapes around me or little squares and swirls.

I've also seen a guy by me. I don't know who it is. I think it might be him. He doesn't talk. It's just like there's another person next to me.

Wiremu: How tall is this person?

Tangi: He's really tall. (indicating taller than her)

Wiremu: That much taller than you?

Tangi: Everyone's taller than me!

Wiremu: I've seen a lot shorter than you!

Tangi: He pats my shoulder. At least he used to when I was little.

Allister: So it's the same fella?

Tangi: Yeah.

Allister: You said you could remember it when you were nine.

Tangi: Yeah, I used to climb trees or play kicks with the ball and he'd come with me. Yeah, I can hear him saying, 'Eh!' He's saying, 'Yeah, that's right.'

Wiremu: Tangi, this person that you see, is he the same age all the time or did he grow up with you?

Tangi: He grew up with me. But he still has the same face. It's kind of weird. His body is taller but his face is the same. In some ways I like him but in some ways I don't.

Wiremu: Is he the one telling you to kill people?

Tangi: Yeah. I like the feeling it gives me even though it's really mental.

Wiremu: Of him being around or the feeling of wanting to kill people?

Tangi: Wanting to kill people.

Allister: That often happens when you're angry, eh?

Tangi: Sometimes not angry. Sometimes it just comes up and then I just restrain myself from doing anything.

Wiremu: I don't see you as an angry person. You look lovely. So where's the angry side of you?

Tangi: It doesn't like to come out with people like you and Allister. It only likes to come out when I'm alone. I don't like being around people. When I'm in class and by myself, I just sit on the desk and the other me will come out. Then I just stick with my work and listen to my music.

Wiremu: You must have heaps of friends, though, because you're part of kapahaka, eh?

Tangi: I have trust issues with friends, like, they're my friends but I don't count them as friends.

At this point Jade joins the session. Tangi tells Jade about her Nan being present at the beginning of the session. Wiremu then asks about her artwork and reminds Tangi that he is keen to see her Hinenuitepō sketches and paintings. Wiremu talks about Tangi finding a way to bring Hinenuitepō back to Hinengaro and Hinetītama, and Tangi interrupts him to explain that she has already begun to do this. Wiremu then speaks about a link that he sees between creativity and spiritual matters.

Wiremu: There are certain things that go along with creativity in te ao wairua. I see lots of young people who are not only very creative, they also have this spiritual awareness.

Jade: Is it something about the mind being more open?

Wiremu: Yeah, it's a portal. Because you're reaching out and grabbing your creativity from somewhere. So it goes beyond a mere natural realm, it goes into a spiritual realm. And sometimes if that doorway is slightly ajar because something has gone in and an obstacle is stopping it from closing, that may prevent you from being selective about what you see and hear and experience. So other things can then come through that doorway.

Now Wiremu realises that he needs to leave the interview because he has a plane to catch.

Wiremu: I'd just like to ask you a question, because I've got to go soon. If I'm to karakia for you to remove that thing, that person that walks alongside you most of the time, I need your permission. Because I can definitely can get that person out. But I have to have your permission to do it. You know, when he tells you to 'kill someone', I don't consider that to be very nice. But that's just my feeling. And like I say, I don't see that in you. I can't see that killing thing, that anger in the Tangi that I see before me. So I was actually inviting that person to get angry while I was about, but as you say, they hide.

Tangi: Yeah, they hide.

Wiremu: So how do you feel about being told to kill people?

While Wiremu has been speaking there has been a marked change in Tangi's āhua (demeanour). Whereas before this she has been very engaged in the interview and quite spontaneous in her responses, suddenly she is hunched over and not looking at us, and her voice has become barely audible.

Tangi: I don't know. I've got a ringing in my ear.

Wiremu: It's okay.

Allister: Tangi, when you and I met up last time and we were talking about Wiremu, it was as if something was giving you a hard time. Is that happening now as well?

(Pause. Tangi is silent, sitting hunched over with her hands over her ears.)

Allister: I could see that you wanted to meet with Wiremu but then, suddenly, it was like something was giving you a hard time about it.

Tangi: Yeah. Ahh!

Wiremu: Then I'm being successful.

Allister: So, I'm getting the sense that you're saying that this fits with some kind of spiritual thing that's happening?

Wiremu: Yes, it's partly to do with her creativity. These things, when they are in danger of being dislodged, usually cause some kind of . . .

Allister: . . . havoc?

Wiremu: Yeah. Because they don't want to leave. Which excites me quite a bit, because it confirms that there is something there and . . .

Allister: . . . something can be done about it?

Wiremu: Yes.

Allister: Tangi, you might need some time to think about the question Wiremu just raised with you. This is a huge thing. This is like a companion that you've had for a long time, and so sometimes young people can worry they'll feel lonely.

Wiremu: Mmm. That's why I asked about the friends.

Allister: Does that make sense Tangi?

Tangi: (silence)

Allister: Wiremu, you'll be back in three days' time. So Tangi, maybe you can think about it over the weekend and we can meet with Wiremu when he returns on Monday.

Third Session with Wiremu

At the beginning of the session three days later, Tangi opens up her sketchbook. She shows us a sketch of a beautiful baby, cradled in the hair of his mother. Tangi explains that the baby in her drawing is Māui.[2] Wiremu comments that even though Māui's mother, Taranga, lost her baby, Māui is protected by her hair. Tangi says that her own mother frequently gets uncomfortable about Tangi drawing babies and talking about babies. Her mother worries that this could drag Tangi down again.

Wiremu: What they say is that something dies in order for something to grow. And I don't think we should ever forget that. My girl just lost her pepe (baby) about four months ago. We had a bit of a kōrero about it. And we said to her, no matter what, your pepe is in a good place. And in your case, your art keeps that pepe in a good place.

Tangi: How did you know?

Wiremu: Oh, sorry! I'm supposed to know some of those things.

Tangi: I like it when you figure these things out.

Wiremu: Keeping pepe alive in your art is not a bad thing. It keeps your pepe safe. Otherwise, there would be more of a loss. This way, you are honouring baby and keeping baby around you, beside you.

Allister: Because sometimes you've felt like your baby is still around you, eh?

Tangi: (in a very quiet voice) I don't call him by that. I usually call him 'black thing'. But he actually has another name.

Wiremu: What's pepe's name?

Tangi: Atarangi.

Wiremu: Oh, that's a beautiful name. It means heavenly light. Atarangi, yeah.

Tangi: M-hmm. It doesn't feel right saying it.

Wiremu: Ko te kōpū o te ao. The first thing you see in the light is te atarangi, and Kōpū, the morning star. They come together. Atarangi is the heavens lighting up at dawn.

Tangi: I don't like saying it because I haven't told Mum yet. She doesn't like me talking about the baby like this.

Wiremu: Has she had an explanation about this? Maybe she thinks it might be harmful for you.

Wiremu then suggests that it would be good to include Tangi's mother in the next session. At this point I steer the conversation towards the question that Wiremu put to Tangi three days before. I ask Wiremu to talk a bit about what was on his mind when he put that question to Tangi.

Wiremu: Well, yes, I did think about that again over the weekend. This person has been a friend to you when there haven't been any other friends around. The only thing that would worry me would be if a friend like this was suggesting that you hurt other people or hurt yourself. I don't want to separate you from a good friend. But if I had a friend who was telling me to go kill someone, then I would question about whether they were really my friend. I think any of us would. Because the thing is you are very talented, you're gifted, you've got art and stuff to do, you can't go round acting out that thing of, it just so happens that one day you feel like killing someone. It'd be such a waste! You know what I mean? You might even reach the NZ Black Sticks and be in the next Olympics. You've got hockey practice tonight after this, haven't you?

Anyway this has been on my mind most of the weekend. I've been thinking about it, worrying about it. That was all. What do you think, girl?

(Pause)

Tangi: Does anyone have a pen?

I hand her a pen and a sheet of paper, and Tangi takes some time to write a sentence on the paper. She then hands it to Wiremu. Wiremu looks at the message and then places it on the table in front of us. Silently he stands and moves around behind Tangi. Then he speaks.

Wiremu: Tangi, I'm taking it from your note that I now have permission to karakia for you. So I will do that karakia now and then we will see how things are for you over the next few days.

Wiremu stands behind Tangi and commences his karakia in te reo Māori. He speaks firmly and emphatically and is directing his energy at a point just behind Tangi. At one point he clicks his fingers in a commanding fashion on that precise spot.

After this there is silence, and then after some time Tangi leaves the room to ring her mother to pick her up.

The Next Six Months

The voice returned once, some weeks later, for one day, but Tangi said she ignored it and it disappeared. Aside from that, for the first time in many years she was not troubled by her voice. Initially this seemed strange and lonely for her. However, she soon got used to it and threw herself into creative pursuits, especially painting. For her final art exam that year, her painting of Hinenuitepō, entitled 'Ki Te Ao Marama' (Into the World of Light) got top marks.

Tangi's occasional spiritual experiences persisted. She would see her brown thing and her white thing. She would sometimes see people who had passed on, but these experiences seemed quite ordinary to her and were in no way troubling. Although I had advised her to continue with her medication treatment,

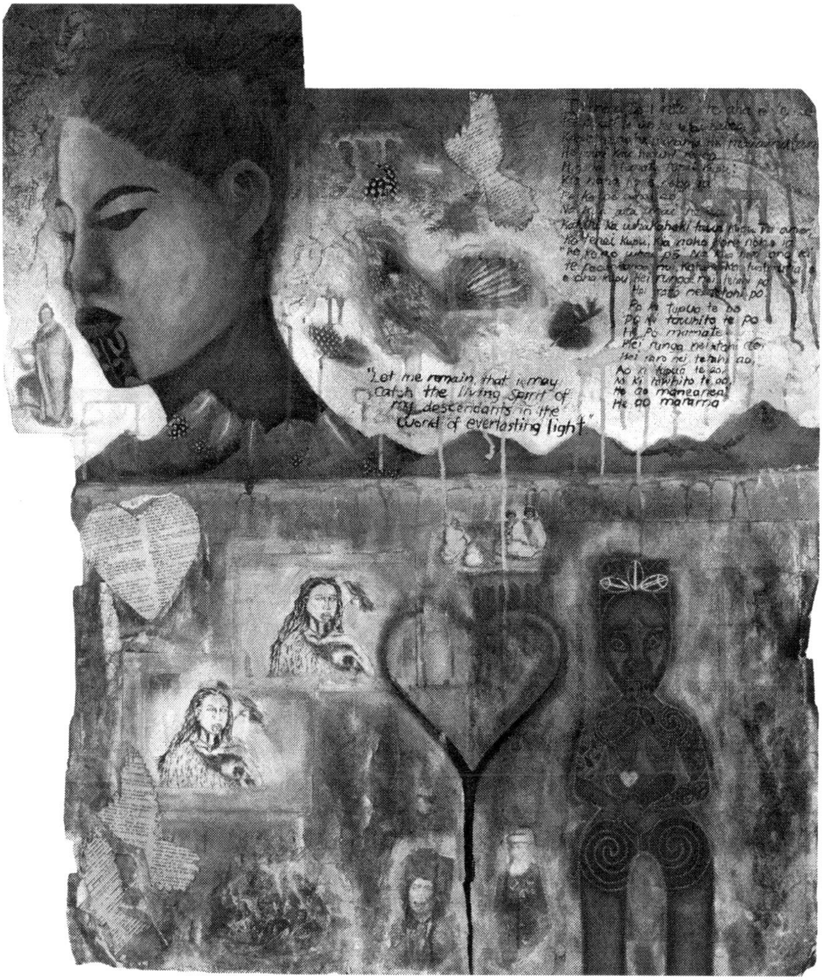
"Let me remain that i may
Catch the living Spirit of
my descendants in the
World of everlasting light"

FIGURE 7.1 Tangi's painting "Ki Te Ao Marama" (Into the World of Light) which depicts Hinenuitepō (bottom right) and Hinetītama (top left)

because she was feeling so well after seeing Wiremu, she had stopped the risperidone.

Six months later it was the summer holidays. Tangi moved in with her partner and his family. She felt well supported and made plans to return to school to finish off some final credits in order to pursue a degree in fine arts, which she hoped might provide a foundation for further training in tā moko (the art of Māori tattooing). She found a job working evening shifts at a local store so that she could contribute financially to her partner's household. However, before long she had some new disturbing experiences.

Tangi

The first thing that happened was that I started hearing several different voices. They were mostly male but not the one that had always been with me before. It freaked me out because I couldn't see them and I felt like I was going crazy.

A week later I first saw this shadowy group of people. The voices seemed to come from that group. The person who stood out for me was a woman. I could see her clearly, although I knew that others wouldn't be able to see her. Her hair was blonde and her eyes were black. She looked Pākehā. She walked really upright. Her skin and clothes were grey. She had a bonnet on her head and was wearing olden-day clothes, perhaps from the 1800s. She had black high-heeled shoes with socks on. Sometimes she wore a long skirt and other times a very short skirt. I was surprised to see that she seemed to be wearing a corset. Sometimes she was alone. Other times she was surrounded by those dark figures. When I saw her at school she was mixed in with some students and I could tell she wasn't a flesh-and-blood person when I saw them walk through her. Once at Koro's place, Tama growled at the spot where I could see her black shoes. I notice the cat comes close to me when she is around.

Allister

Although initially the voices seemed benign, before long a voice would encourage Tangi to act on her angry feelings. Sometimes this voice would tell her to kill or harm the people she was angry with at the time. Once, when Tangi became upset and angry with her partner, a voice goaded her into grabbing a kitchen knife and threatening him with it. She felt very alarmed and contacted our service, asking to be seen urgently.

At our appointment Tangi spoke of the voices and figures that she had seen. She drew a picture of the figures and the way they appeared to her. As her psychiatrist, I also felt alarmed about what she had described. In particular, her description of voices telling her to kill and harm others, combined with Tangi threatening her partner with a knife, suggested to me that this was a high-risk situation that needed to be addressed urgently.[3] In addition to the voices, it was clear that she was feeling more and more depressed, fearing that she was going crazy as she struggled to make sense of her experiences. Her sleep had been poor for weeks because she was working late and getting up early for school. She was unable to concentrate and had lost motivation for her art. She revealed that she had stopped her fluoxetine (antidepressant) treatment three months before, as she had been feeling so well. We were concerned about the serious risk she posed to her partner and others, so we encouraged Tangi to consider admission to a local youth crisis respite house. She agreed, but with some trepidation.

Because of Wiremu's previous intervention and the relief it had given Tangi, I was curious to know what his view would be about the situation. However,

Wiremu was out of town and I knew he wouldn't be returning for some weeks. In light of the distressing voices, her depression symptoms, and her previous serious depressive episode, I recommended to Tangi that we restart her antidepressant medication to address her depression and start antipsychotic medication to reduce the intensity of the voices and help her sleep better. She was keen to proceed with both these options.

I anticipated that a week in Headspace—our local youth respite house—with the friendly staff and relaxed atmosphere there would be just the tonic for Tangi. And it would remove her from the stress of the intensity of her intimate relationship, as well as from school and work pressures.

However, when I next met with her she was even more distressed.

Tangi

Even though I was seeing the lady and the shadowy group before, at Headspace it became much more full-on. Frequently I would see her and the group of figures standing out on the balcony. I could see a big brick building with a clock just behind them, which no one else could see. She was in the middle, with the others making a circle around her. They felt negative. They were always just black shadows. She seemed to be using them to scare me. The thing that really freaked me out was the screeching: it was high-pitched and got more and more intense. It made me really scared and I didn't feel safe at Headspace. I felt scared because it seemed like there were no barriers—they could just come in whenever they wanted. My mind wasn't in a good place. My barriers weren't working.

Allister

At this time Tangi spoke about thoughts of wishing she was dead. She felt alarmed by her own impulses to kill herself. She had little hope of any relief from the screeching that was tormenting her. She wanted to leave Headspace and didn't want to go home. When I offered admission to our local adolescent inpatient psychiatry unit, with an air of resignation she agreed.

Her first hospital stay lasted 10 days. Over this time the voices and screeching reduced in intensity. Tangi said it seemed like there was a wall between her and them. With the relief from this onslaught and encouragement to attend to the various stressful things in her life, Tangi felt that her mood and suicidal thoughts were lifting and she was keen to be discharged. She quit her part-time job and reduced the demands of school. She resolved to attend to important matters in her relationship with her boyfriend.

After leaving hospital Tangi remained optimistic in her outlook; however, despite the antipsychotic treatment she was on, she noticed a steady increase in the intensity of the voices and the distressing screeching sounds. She would frequently see glimpses of the woman's black shoes or the edge of her skirt. At times she could feel an unpleasant presence and she felt sure that this was the same apparition.

When I next saw her she asked after Wiremu. We discussed her recent experiences and weighed up factors that supported a diagnosis of psychosis and factors that suggested she might have a spiritual problem, and we even considered if it could be a combination of both. Wiremu was due to visit in two weeks, and Tangi was very keen to see him. When I offered to ring him and enquire about his views on her situation, she enthusiastically agreed. I suggested that we could ask Wiremu to do a karakia for her, and she was equally adamant that she would like that.

Later that day I phoned Wiremu. I explained that I was ringing on behalf of Tangi and that she had been troubled by experiences in which she would see a woman with white hair who looked grey in appearance. Wiremu interrupted me to relay an incident from two nights before. He had been sitting on his bed late that evening and suddenly, above him, there appeared 'a very freaky lady'. He told me she had white or silver hair, and her mouth was wide open as if she was yelling or howling at him, although he heard no noise. She was looming over him in a threatening manner, and her hands were in a claw-like posture as if she was about to try to scratch him with her fingernails. After recovering from his initial fright Wiremu demanded that she leave in no uncertain terms. He said that the whole experience had lasted about 20 seconds. At the time he had been unsure of how to make sense of this unwanted 'visit'.

I was taken aback by Wiremu's description, and even more nonplussed when he said that he was now certain that this was the same 'lady' that Tangi had been dealing with. He was delighted to do a karakia to assist Tangi that same evening. He was sure that it would be possible to deal with this 'lady' as she was 'really not nice'.

My head still reeling, I rang Tangi to relay Wiremu's news. In my own mind it was hard to fathom how Wiremu's experience, 500 kilometres away, could have anything to do with Tangi—yet he seemed so sure about it. As soon as I told Tangi, she was immediately certain that the figure Wiremu had seen was the same woman. At the moment when I described what Wiremu had told me, she said she suddenly had a clear picture in her mind of the face that he had seen and she was sure it was the same woman who had been tormenting her. I could hear the relief in her voice: 'Wiremu has seen her too. I'm not crazy!' She recounted a frightening dream about this woman early on the morning of the same day as Wiremu's experience; that evening she was feeling particularly tense and anxious, and had a strong feeling that the woman was in her immediate presence. This unpleasant feeling became more intense as the evening wore on until she could hardly bear it. Finally it subsided by about 10 p.m. Tangi said she was not at all surprised that this was the time when Wiremu had his experience. She was sure the experiences were related and believed the apparition had been trying to scare Wiremu.

At our subsequent appointment Tangi described what happened after my phone call to her:

> Sometime during the evening, perhaps it was about nine o'clock, suddenly the screeching began to get really intense. I could feel something quite evil around me and it felt like she was scratching me and clawing me around my face. I could see glimpses of her shoes and skirt, as I had before. Although I felt quite scared when it happened I also had confidence that Wiremu could help me. After half an hour of intense screeching, her voice began to fade and gradually disappeared altogether.

Over the ensuing period, there was no more of the screeching voice or any other voices. However, at that end of that time Tangi became very distressed when her boyfriend, who had been struggling to make sense of her recent distress and experiences, initiated a break-up of their relationship. This loss, as well as the loss of the support that she had experienced from his family, left her feeling suddenly bereft. During this crisis, Tangi's intense impulses to end her life and harm herself returned. Reluctantly she agreed to a further admission to the adolescent inpatient psychiatry unit for her safety.

Although the voices didn't return immediately, Tangi's hospital stay was a tumultuous time for her, eventually lasting two months. 'The lady' returned to torment her with screeching at times, and she described several other voices. Tangi's psychiatrist on the inpatient unit was of the view that the experiences she was describing were consistent with a quite severe psychotic illness. Nevertheless, Wiremu and I visited Tangi on a number of occasions, and Wiremu reasserted his view that many of her experiences were likely to be spiritual in origin. Tangi's hospital psychiatrists worked closely with us as her community team, and we had a number of involved conversations about her puzzling experiences and symptoms. We persisted in considering the psychiatric and cultural explanations for her situation alongside each other.

Tangi remained confused about whether her experiences were spiritual in origin, but she was always pleased to see Wiremu, and she seemed reassured when he would confirm the presence of this 'lady' near to her and relieved when he was able to locate 'her' in space in the same spot that she could identify. Tangi was persevering with medication treatment, including fluoxetine and her antipsychotic medication, which was changed to aripiprazole. However, it was unclear if moderate doses of this antipsychotic agent were making any appreciable difference to the intensity of the voices she was describing, and later this medication was changed to quetiapine, another antipsychotic treatment, which would also assist her with sleep difficulties.

During several of Wiremu's sessions with Tangi on the adolescent unit, he reaffirmed that he was still able to detect the presence of a female entity next to Tangi, and he remained convinced that it was the same one that had 'visited' him that night in his home 500 kilometres away. However, Wiremu now explained to Tangi that it was necessary for her to make the decision to take charge of these entities that were impinging on her. It would not be easy initially, but he was confident that she could take this step. He was also sure that focusing on her gifts, including her art and sport, was likely to be important in this quest.

Meanwhile, Tangi's Māori trainee psychiatrist introduced her to a local tā moko artist, and he invited her to visit his studio. Her skill as an artist and her passion for tā moko made an impression on this tohunga (expert), and she became a regular visitor to his studio. For Tangi, this was a dream come true. When she left the unit, her mother arranged space in their small flat for Tangi to return home to live with her, her partner, and Tangi's brother. Despite her mother's initial trepidation because of Tangi's previous threatening behaviour, over time they were able to rebuild their trust in one another, and their mother–daughter relationship slowly but surely flourished.

Wiremu

After the First Three Sessions

It was in our second session together that I gradually gained a clearer impression of the 'thing' that was hanging around Tangi. During our kōrero it seemed like this entity was trying to fade right into the background. At first I wasn't sure it was there, but when I was asking Tangi's permission to do a karakia for her, her eyes moved around really fast. At that point I knew the entity was there and I got quite excited, I thought 'Whoa!' By this time, the thing was retreating and communicating with her. Then, all of a sudden, she blocked off her ears. It was hiding away and telling her 'Don't be any part of this, don't listen. I don't wanna hear that.'

This was really difficult for Tangi—I'm surprised she didn't scream or yell. I think she must have wanted to work with me because often in those moments these things can cause a person to scream and swear, 'Get the . . .!' They get abusive, they throw things around. I knew it had the influence to do that to her. So I decided to proceed quietly. I thought that the short entity that I saw was the same as the tall one she talked about. I knew this gremlin had been around her for a long time, and she might not be sure if she wanted to get rid of it. So I told her, 'I have to go now, but I have seen this "thing" that's with you, and if you want me to get rid of it, I can do that. You need to really decide if that's what you want. If you like we can meet up after the weekend.'

That first session was on a Friday. Our next session was on the following Monday, and at that session Tangi had made a decision; however, she couldn't say it out loud. Initially, I didn't see the thing, as I had on the Friday. I knew it was trying to hide. But after a while I saw it in her eyes. When I asked her what she had decided, she hesitated for a while and looked like she wanted to say something but couldn't. She asked for a piece of paper and a pen, and she wrote something down and handed it to me. The note read, 'I can't say it out loud, but I want to get rid of it.' I knew then that she had given me her permission: she was trying to express this without letting the thing stop her or without letting it know that she was communicating with me.

I stood and walked round behind her to karakia for her. At that point I saw her put her fingers in her ears again. It was as if she was trying to block out some of what I was saying in the karakia—or, more likely, the thing was trying to block it out by getting her to do that. Because of that, I asked Te Kaihanga (the creator) to open Tangi's ears so that the thing could hear the authority that was coming. I didn't have to yell or say, 'Get the hell out of here!' I just let Te Kaihanga do it. I knew that the creator could do it much better than I could.

As far as I was concerned, it was out of there, and only she could let it back in. I knew the results would become clear over the next week. I emphasised to Allister and Jade that it would be important to reinforce the fact that she had the mana to be in charge all the time. That would be a way for her to get rid of that thing permanently, if she wanted that.

It interests me that these things can have different appearances to different people. The location can appear to change as well. With Tangi, I could tell it was located within her, and at one point I saw it just beside her. It wasn't a full person I saw. It was only 18 inches high. It had a very small body, but a head about four inches high, with the body fitting the head. The figure I saw was like a doll. During the session I asked Tangi how tall it was, and she said it was taller than her. I asked that because the thing I was seeing wasn't very tall at all. And straight after our session, when she stepped out of the room, she commented to me: 'Gee, you're short!' That really amused me.

At the last session I met Tangi's mother for the first time. It was apparent to me that she needed some help as well. Finding out about Tangi's voices telling her to kill people had been pretty frightening for her. And I picked up that there were past matters that were still troubling her. So I have offered her a time to meet up.

Eight Months Later: The Lady

The night that I had a visit from 'the screeching lady', I was up at my farm near Gisborne. I had arrived home from town in the late evening and it was getting dark. I went to lie back on my bed and—Woom!—this creature came flying straight down at me. It had its arms out, mouth wide open as if it was screaming at me, but there was no sound. It was very ugly, with white hair, very white all over. Looking back, I don't think the message was for me. I wasn't the target. I expect it was trying to scare me, but I'm more than positive that Tangi was the target. I wonder if it was connected to Tangi's aspiration to become a tā moko artist. That's a very sacred art, it's tapu. This creature was there to hinder her journey. If you are working towards doing good things for people, then these things have a way of targeting you, to try to change your mind or scare you off your track.

Session on the Unit

About six weeks later I saw Tangi on the rangatahi (adolescent) unit. She was still hearing the screeching lady, and as far as the doctors were concerned it looked quite psychotic. While she was telling me about the screeching and yelling that was still going on, I detected that presence in the room. It seemed to be behind her left shoulder, looming over her. It was like it had talons coming from the fingers of both its hands, ready to strike. So I went over to sit by her. And when Tangi asked if I could feel that this lady was there, I said 'Yes.' After that I put my left arm around her shoulders so that if there was going to be a strike, it would strike my arm first. My arm felt cold, clammy, and unpleasant where the anger and the venom of that thing was hitting it. Tangi said my arm felt cold and frozen, even though the room itself wasn't cold.

By this time, I knew it was important for Tangi to develop her own ways to spiritually defend herself. I believe the person I'm trying to help needs to do 75 percent of the work—otherwise, I would have to come in every time someone needs to have a karakia. I would rather do myself out of a job. It was time for Tangi to develop her own spiritual immune system so that she herself could respond whenever she was faced with some spiritual bug or virus, even when I wasn't there. This was about her mana. If she could do this, then she would have authority over her circumstances.

In the Whānau Room in the Adolescent Psychiatry Unit

In a later meeting on the unit, which her whānau attended, Tangi was hunched over, feeling very cold. That thing was still there. I could see that she hadn't yet built up that self-defence—she had yet to become a seasoned fighter, if I can put it that way. But she was getting there. I knew that every day that she stayed well and worked at what she was passionate about, she would get better and stronger. I wanted to encourage her to find a way to get rid of it. If she had been in real danger then I would have had to remove it again myself, but by this time, I needed to hold back so that she would have the chance to use her own mana to deal with it and then start to build up her own confidence.

A while ago, some months after Tangi had been discharged from the adolescent unit, we met at Te Whare Mārie. She had been having a hard time that week and hearing the voice quite intensely, but I could see that she was getting stronger. This time, when we were wrapping up the session, it was important that Tangi was the one to do our karakia. She used a karakia that had been given to her by her tā moko kaiako (teacher). And you could see afterwards that she felt good about that—that her confidence was growing.

Since then when I have spoken to Tangi, the lady that was tormenting her for so many months has very little power in her life. Tangi has taken charge and she is now the boss of it. That thing will be of no consequence shortly; it won't have any power to be dictating to her what she has to do. But, of course, she is such a spiritual person that, more than likely, she will continue to have spiritual experiences.

As far as I'm concerned, this has been a much more profound learning experience for her than if I just did a karakia and got rid of it again until the next spiritual germ came along. And this learning is a lot to do with her relationship with her tā moko teacher and his constant presence and the work that he does to whakamana her (strengthen her mana) every day. She is very lucky to work with a tā moko tohunga of his standing. He is very mindful of the spiritual implications of his art. If you are practising tā moko, this is a particular kind of journey that could attract a particular kind of spiritual germ. So she has a great teacher to help protect her with that.

In other parts of her life she has also been healing some old wounds. She and her mother have worked on healing their relationship since she left the unit. All these things have been important in her building up that mana in her life.

Nine Months after Tangi's Final Admission to Hospital

When I think about Tangi's experiences over the last 11 months since the screeching lady entered her life, I wonder how we can understand her having such experiences even after our previous sessions and banishing the black thing. Well, as I said at the time, once the black thing had been removed, it was up to Tangi what she would let back in. It reminds me of autumn, when the leaves are lying on the ground and the wind is blowing. If Tangi opens the door to her house, the leaves can get blown in. We might go in and sweep all those leaves out again with a broom and shut the door. And they stay outside while the door is closed. But if Tangi opens that door again and the wind's blowing that way, the leaves will blow in again, perhaps more than before. If Tangi were to partake in any substances that are no good for her, then that door can get wedged open. If that happens, she may not be able to control what leaves are coming through that doorway.

When Tangi had her setback and was being harassed by the screeching lady, I still knew it was a spiritual problem. I was confident about that because I had an experience with the screaming woman that I was sure was related to what Tangi had seen. If you ask me, the chances of us both having an identical experience like that in such a timeframe must be a million to one! Even before that I could see that it was wairua stuff going on for her. However, I was asking the question: What had happened for her door to be flung open like that? I knew that she was affected by the relationships around her and the losses she'd been through. Then she was rocked by her relationship break-up. Being in such a vulnerable emotional state could have a similar effect to taking drugs like cannabis. It could open that door and allow something problematic to find its way in.

When I saw Tangi this week, I could tell that she is making great progress. There has been a marked change from how she was when I saw her during her time in hospital. Of course, it's still possible she could have another setback. But she's getting a grip on what she wants to do in her life and how she might achieve it. She is also quite content not being in an intimate relationship. I'm happy to hear that. I wouldn't begrudge her having a relationship, but I wouldn't like to see her get into a relationship at this point that could negatively affect her well-being. I wouldn't like to see anything that might hinder her progress on her journey to be a tā moko artist.

Tangi

Ten Days after the Third Session

In the last 10 days since seeing Wiremu and since his karakia for me, I haven't heard the voice at all. It's weird and lonely, but good in a way. I can't remember the last time that I've had 10 days without this voice in my life—it's been there for such a long time.

My first memories of seeing things are from when I was about four years old. They started coming to me at nighttime and hiding in the corner. Over time I got used to that. Then in my primary years, when I was around eight, I was getting bullied a lot, and this fella would hang around with me at school. I didn't know his name, so I used to call him 'my little friend'. He was my best friend that nobody else could see. Because I knew that I could see and hear things that others couldn't, I felt different and tended to isolate myself. He would encourage me to be more antisocial. At times I would have no friends except him, and he seemed to want it that way. In a way he was kind of evil, but he was also cool. However, sometimes he would make me do things that were really not good—things that I normally wouldn't have thought of doing. For example, one time he got really angry at me for patting a little kitten. He told me, 'You better kill him', which I did. After that I felt terrible. That was when I was eight and that was a really bad experience with him.

The main voice I hear has always been the same male voice. He would identify himself only as my 'friend'. I accepted it because I was used to seeing things. He would be there at night. Sometimes I wouldn't talk to him, but he would be there every night talking to me.

In these last 10 days it's been such a relief because I haven't had the urges to kill people. I haven't had anyone telling me to do anything stupid—things like telling me to smoke weed or cut myself. Previously the voice was often telling me things like 'Why don't you hurt that person for calling you that?' or 'Why is he staring at you like that? Go find out.' I was sniffing petrol to try to block him out. I don't know why, but it would block my mind from hearing him for half an hour; but then, after it wore off, he would just get worse. Sometimes smoking weed would also block him out for a short time.

The voice would only be positive in my life when I was by myself, when no one else was around. When someone else was around, he would get angry.

When I was surrounded by friends, it would be worse—it was like he was jealous. When I was going through really hard times, the voice used to tell me I deserved it, but he said he would always be there for me; no one else would be there like he was.

I never spoke about the voice before because I thought Allister and Jade would stick me in hospital. I thought they would think I was crazy. But I was also scared that I was crazy and sometimes I would call myself 'mental'.

Since Wiremu did the karakia, my life has felt boring in both a good and a bad way. On the good side, my painting has been going well. I've done what Wiremu suggested, incorporating Hinetītama into my artwork. After the termination, I missed a whole year of my art. I just couldn't be bothered. I was so sad that I just couldn't face it. After meeting Jade and Allister, I started drawing and painting again.

I have always been interested in death and what happens after life. Recently my art teacher asked us to retell a legend. I chose to do Hinenuitepō and the fantail. I've always been interested in Hinenuitepō. I like her because she is all dark, not evil, but just dark. That's what she means to me. It's because of my interest in death and the spiritual side. And she's a lady—not like Hades who is a dude and he's ugly! In the Western traditions they are all dudes! But in te ao Māori it's mixed, and I like that.

The depression influenced me to focus on her because at that time I wanted to die. Actually I didn't really want to end my life, but I wanted to experience death. So the depression made me think about death more every day and especially at nighttime. And so when I heard about Hinenuitepō I was very interested. I asked my art teacher if I could do Hinenuitepō as one of my main characters. Six weeks later I met Wiremu. When Wiremu began talking about Hinenuitepō, I was surprised. Later on, when he suggested that I should begin to bring her back from the darkness to the light, I was blown away by that idea and how well it fit with what I was focused on in my art. It made sense to me.

These days, thinking about the termination doesn't feel so painful for me. When other people talk about it, I feel a twinge, but I can just shake it off. I don't dwell on it anymore because Mum always says, 'You can't take it back.' I think I've got that in my head now. It was always hard for me to forgive myself, but I think I've been able to do that now.

It's hard to remember how difficult things were for me a month ago. I've only got glimpses of that time now and I know that the voice was giving me a very hard time. Now it's hard to think about it, perhaps because I feel so different. My mood is definitely better.

Nine Months after Tangi's Final Admission to Hospital

Meeting Wiremu for the first time was nerve-wracking, but I knew it could help me. Before I met him, I was hoping that he wouldn't know anything about me, so that we could be on the same level or at least open-minded about each other.

During that first meeting, it wasn't long before I could feel something suggesting to me that he was trying to read my mind. And at the same time I was trying to do it to him, and it felt like a kind of mind battle! And I talked to Wiremu about this. I said, 'What are you doing?' and he said, 'Well, what are you doing?' and I responded, 'Oh nothing!' After that we both started laughing, because both of us knew that we had made that connection.

Mana, the Black Thing, and Karakia

That first time we met, Wiremu brought up 'mana'. He explained how if you build up your mana, it can be like a wall. By gradually building up that wall, it can help protect you from negative spiritual things and keep you sane.

In the second session with Wiremu, he saw something and asked if he could do a karakia for me. It took me a while to come up with an answer. I had the other guy telling me, 'Stay away from Wiremu.' He couldn't stand Wiremu at all! So he would beat me up mentally about Wiremu and scream in my ears. I would block my ears and try to get rid of him.

In the third session, I decided in my mind that I wanted the karakia. I realised it was impossible for me to say out loud: 'Yes, I want this karakia.' Somehow he was stopping me from saying it. I couldn't think clearly. I had an awful feeling of pressure at the back of my head, my left shoulder, and on my back. It was getting really cold and heavy. Somehow that was familiar to me from times when he was angry over the years. So I did the only thing I could. I wrote a note to Wiremu to let him know that I would like him to do the karakia. After that, Wiremu stood at the back of me. He was holding my hand, and the intensity of the black thing got even worse and he was telling me to kill everyone in the room. And the pressure to hurt them, or hurt myself, was so intense I couldn't bear it any longer.

Suddenly I heard this big ugly screech and it was gone. That was it. He returned on and off for a couple of days. After that he disappeared.

Wiremu and the Screeching Lady

Six months later, this new lady suddenly appeared in my life—I have described her in detail earlier in this chapter. After a few weeks she became so unpleasant, it felt like she was trying to torture me. The worst thing was the screeching. Eventually I realised she was quite evil. There was a bad feeling that feeds onto you and it changes your personality. Dealing with her was really hard. She would literally come up to me and scratch and hurt me in other ways. She ended up putting me in hospital for a while and continued torturing me for some weeks.

After my first time in hospital I met up with Allister and he offered to ring Wiremu about it. Later that day he called me back. He explained that Wiremu had had an experience with a lady, and I knew straight away that it was her. As soon as Allister said what Wiremu had seen, the exact scene came straight to me.

What he saw and what he felt at that moment were crystal clear to me: this lady was showing me what she did to Wiremu. I knew that she was dangerous, but through this time I was very confused about whether I was dealing with schizophrenia or something spiritual. But at that moment, having Wiremu go through that experience helped me a great deal. It reaffirmed what he had been telling me, that I have this gift. I didn't have psychosis. It was that confirmation that I'm okay and I'm not alone. I had always felt so alone in my life.

Recent Experiences

In recent times things have been going well for me. I've got my head much more sussed out. I have been slowly sorting out my feelings towards myself. I have been gradually accepting who I am as a person and how all these full-on experiences fit in with who I am.

I continue to have spiritual experiences every day. Some days it can happen right through the day. At times they get really rowdy, and I can't tell why. I realise now this is just the nature of what I call wairua, the spirits. They have their little outbursts and might even seem to take it out on me, but I just carry on with what I'm doing. Those outbursts can be in the physical realm, like when they fling a door open, or they bang a wall. I might hear tapping sounds or hear footsteps when no one is there, or occasionally a screech or a scream. Sometimes I get a distinct feeling that someone has touched me, even though there is no one physically there. I have gotten used to it now.

I have always had feelings about certain places or people—for example, I can get a clear feeling that a person is not good. I have a strong impulse to stay away from them. With some places, I will instinctively know that I shouldn't go there—something or somebody is telling me 'no', like a protection.

I frequently see figures darting past out of the corner of my eye. The figures look human. Often I can't see their faces clearly but I may see them inside my head. They're like little cheeky goblins, running around in the edges of my vision.

I often see auras around people or around places. I often have dreams about things I don't understand, but sometime later they come true. They are like prediction dreams. So I take more notice of my dreams these days.

For me now, things have quietened down, they are easier to ignore than they were. But I still know that they are there.

Allister

Hearing voices has been reported in many civilisations over the ages. Socrates, at his trial prior to his death in 399 BC, reported hearing a voice throughout his life guiding him to avoid certain actions, which he viewed as a positive influence (Escher & Romme, 2010). Joan of Arc used her experience of voices to assist her successful military strategy in 1429; however, when she was captured her descriptions of voices were used against her as evidence of witchcraft. Descriptions of hearing voices have been common in religious traditions, with well-known examples in Christianity such as Hildegard of Bingen, Teresa of Avila, and Francis of Assisi. In indigenous societies, there are accounts of hearing voices in many traditions; often they are interpreted as messages from spirits. Black Elk of the Oglala Sioux recalled his first experience of hearing a voice at the age of nine, and later viewed it as heralding his calling as a medicine man (Neihardt, 1988). John Fire Lame Deer, a Lakota medicine man, gave a similar account (Lame Deer & Erdoes, 1972). Odi Oquosa, a Nigerian healer living in England, described hearing voices from an early age that guided him in his later vocation as a shaman (Romme et al., 2009). There are descriptions of hearing voices from other healers in South America and West Africa (Kopenawa & Albert, 2013; Somé, 1994).

There are numerous accounts of Māori healers and prophets hearing voices. Te Kooti Arikirangi Te Turuki described hearing voices on several occasions in 1867, and the Ringatū Church dates its origin to the revelations from those experiences (Binney, 1995). Tahupōtiki Wiremu Rātana experienced a number of voices and visions, beginning in 1918, that prompted him to begin his healing work and later to establish the Rātana Church (Newman, 2009). Māori healer Hohepa Kereopa described an example of his own experiences:

> Some people say that they can hear voices in their heads, telling them to do certain things. For me, I don't hear that sort of voice. Any voice I do hear, I can pinpoint a body to it—someone from the past, and I even see them . . . One time, I heard someone behind me, and I saw an old lady wearing a cardigan over her shoulders, and she said that everything was alright. And I thought to myself, 'Now, who wears a cardigan like that?' And then I remembered. It was one of my aunties. And that afternoon, I got the phone call. She had passed away.
>
> *(Moon, 2003: pp. 109–110)*

Simon McCarthy-Jones (2012) points out that there have always existed 'two jostling discourses' about hearing voices: one in which these experiences are viewed as pathological, exemplified in modern times by the biomedical model; the other in which such experiences are viewed as spiritual and meaningful. A detailed exposition of the nuances of this debate is beyond the scope of this chapter; however, in my training in medicine and psychiatry, naturally the emphasis was strongly on the biomedical model. After all, the concept of the biological basis of psychosis had been established from the 1890s onwards, first articulated by Emil Kraepelin, the German psychiatrist who developed his classification of mental illnesses and described the syndrome of dementia praecox, the forerunner of what is now called schizophrenia (Sadock & Sadock, 2005.) Further compelling evidence seemed to come from the discovery of medications such as chlorpromazine in the 1950s which, for the first time, suppressed distressing hallucinations, delusions, and other psychotic symptoms, and every so often appeared to extinguish them altogether.

All doctors, in their training, will have seen people suffering from a severe psychotic illness that is acutely distressing, disabling, and life threatening, who have improved considerably after a few weeks of modern antipsychotic medication treatment. They will have seen someone with acute delirium experiencing dramatic psychotic symptoms that quite clearly have been caused by an organic brain problem. The recognition of a neurochemical mechanism for the beneficial effect of antipsychotic treatment also appears to be strong evidence that supports the disease model of schizophrenia. Hence, such a discourse in medicine and psychiatry is so dominant that there is little room to question whether there might be such a thing as normally hearing voices or hallucinations, unless they are associated with sleep onset or waking up. In this paradigm, any hallucination is assumed to be a symptom of brain pathology until proven otherwise; and, of course, disproof may be impossible. As a result, someone presenting to a psychiatrist with unexplained, nondistressing voices could be viewed as likely to develop a psychiatric, if not psychotic, illness at a later time. Any patients who do later present with distressing psychotic symptoms help confirm the disease model. Those who don't won't be seen again, and that evidence is lost. In Tangi's situation, she did not meet the criteria for schizophrenia but experienced voices and visions that were very distressing for her during her crisis time.

Population studies since the 1990s have shown that 4 percent of the overall population in a range of Western countries hear voices that would qualify under the psychiatric definition of an auditory hallucination, and two-thirds of those are untroubled by them or may even find them helpful (Romme et al., 2009; Tien, 1991; van Os et al., 2001). Romme et al. have documented accounts from 50 people who heard voices, who recovered from distressing voices and learnt to cope with and change their relationship with their voices, with or without assistance from psychiatric services (Romme et al., 2009). From their research, these authors described three phases of recovery: the initial 'startled' phase, characterised by high anxiety and feeling overwhelmed; the 'organisation' phase in which the person hearing voices becomes interested in the experience and seeks more information; and the 'stabilisation' phase in which the person regains their own confidence, potential, and abilities.

In general terms these three phases seem consistent with Tangi's progress over time. Although Wiremu's intervention after session three seemed to provide immediate relief, the voices and visions that she experienced six months later clearly overwhelmed her ability to cope. Romme et al. (2009) describe the most commonly dispiriting aspects as 'the threats, the feelings of powerlessness and the anxiety of being mad' (p. 1)—and each of these factors certainly seemed to take a toll on Tangi. Later, Wiremu's experience of the 'screeching lady' seemed to give her information that helped her organise her response to it. As she became more confident about her spiritual understanding of the problem, a wide range of factors are likely to have contributed to her 'stabilisation' phase. Ongoing reference to Wiremu's advice and support, low to moderate doses of antipsychotic medication (which is likely to have eased her anxiety and reduced the intensity of her voices), the support of hospital staff and family, and subsequently the relationship with her tā moko teacher all seemed to be important in her recovery process.

As a psychiatrist, I am left wondering about the relative contributions of spirituality, trauma, psychosis, and other explanations such as cannabis use for Tangi's dramatic and distressing experiences. Wiremu's assessment persuaded me that a substantial proportion of her disturbing perceptual experiences could be viewed as a spiritual problem; but it seems to me likely that there has been a contribution from each of these factors.

Ron Coleman (1999) has heard voices since his early adult life and spent 10 years in a psychiatric hospital in his early adulthood with a diagnosis of schizophrenia. He is a strong advocate for the recovery movement and speaks eloquently and humorously about experiences on his path to recovery. He has identified four important components in recovery. First, *involving others*—this can inspire hope and provide support, companionship, and a sense of direction; second, *working on the self* to improve self-esteem and develop confidence, acceptance, and awareness of oneself; third, *making choices*, developing a stronger sense of personal responsibility and finding a purpose in life; and finally, *taking ownership* of one's own voice-hearing experience.

Ron's ideas come from his Scottish cultural perspective; nevertheless, his advice resonates with Wiremu's concepts of mana and building up one's own spiritual authority in relation to disturbing perceptual experiences.

At the time of this writing, it is two years since Tangi was discharged from her second hospital admission. She was discharged from our service nine months ago, as she was happy with her progress and didn't feel a need for anything further from us at that time. The only medication she continues to take is a low dose of quetiapine, prescribed by her family doctor to help her sleep on an as-required basis. There has been no return of her previous depression. She continues to experience voices and visions most days, which she considers to be spiritual in origin. Although occasionally they can become uncomfortable in their intensity, she considers that part and parcel of having a spiritual gift. She is living with a supportive partner and has begun a Māori arts course at a local Māori wānanga or university.

We finish the chapter with Tangi's words on the most helpful elements in her recovery in the first year after her hospital admissions.

Tangi

A number of things have helped me get through my experiences with depression and wairua in the last year. One of these has been my art. I have continued to focus on Hinetītama and Hinenuitepō in my drawing and painting. Bringing back Hine from the darkness to Hinetītama seemed to symbolise the start of my recovery. Other big influences are tā moko—and especially my teacher—as well as the help from Te Whare Mārie. I've learned a lot over the last months and gained experience.

I want to be a tā moko artist and help rangatahi who suffer from mental illness or from the same thing that I do—spiritual experiences that can be very negative. When you are young you may not understand what is going on for you. I think some young people who are having these experiences could be helped by traditional Māori arts like tā moko. Young people may be freaked out by spiritual experiences and think they are weird or have a mental health problem. Then, if doctors don't understand about spiritual experiences and label a young person's spiritual experiences as psychosis, this can add to the problem.

The process of preparing and then getting a moko is healing. When a tā moko is designed for you and then when it is etched onto your skin, it comes to embody, to symbolise who you are. It can depict your beliefs, your whakapapa or genealogy, who you love, and your identity. It often contains your kaitiaki, those ancestors or others who continue to provide you with protection. Once you get your moko on, once you have your kaitiaki printed on you, they are on there permanently. It helps your mana, because it helps you feel proud of who you are and what you have. If you have a gift or a mental illness, it's not going to put you down. You can still do stuff that other people can do.

In the last few months, things have picked up for me. I feel motivated because of my teacher to get out of bed to do tā moko. My mood has been better. I continue to see the screeching lady; however, she doesn't screech. She doesn't annoy me. I see her out of the corner of my eye, walking around or staring, but that's about it. She's a spirit. She seems to like to hang around me, but she doesn't bother me now.

The first few times, Wiremu's karakia was very important for me. But last time we met he asked me to do the karakia. I think he did that because he wants me to be strong enough to deal with these things myself. He was giving me the mana. These days, if Wiremu knows I'm in a bad situation, he's not chasing it away but he's handing it back to me. He wants me to find my own mana. But it's more than just about mana. It's also related to the spirits themselves. He wants me to change my relationship with them. He wants me to be thinking about why they might be annoying me. He wants me to be in charge of that relationship.

Notes

1. These exercises and others that Jade introduced to help Tangi manage strong negative feelings were drawn from a modality known as dialectical behaviour therapy.
2. Māui was a Māori hero who as an infant was set adrift into the sea by his mother, Taranga, wrapped in hair from her tikitiki (topknot)—hence he is sometimes known as Māui-tikitiki-a-Taranga. He was nurtured by ocean spirits until he drifted to land.

3. As described earlier in this chapter, these types of voices are known in psychiatry as command hallucinations and are generally considered a hallmark of a serious psychotic condition.

References

Binney, J. (1995) *Redemption songs: A life of the Nineteenth-Century Maori Leader Te Kooti Arikirangi Te Turuki*. University of Hawai'i Press, Honolulu.

Coleman, R. (1999) *Recovery: An alien concept*. Handsell Publishing, Gloucester.

Escher, S. & Romme, M. (eds) (2010) *Young people hearing voices: What you need to know and what you can do*. PCCS Books, Herefordshire.

Kopenawa, D. & Albert, B. (2013) *The falling sky: Words of a Yanomami Shaman*. Belknap Press, Harvard University Press, Cambridge, MA.

Lame Deer, J.F. & Erdoes, R. (1972) *Lame Deer: Seeker of visions*. Simon & Schuster, New York.

McCarthy-Jones, S. (2012) *Hearing voices: The histories, causes and meanings of auditory verbal hallucinations*. Cambridge University Press, Cambridge.

Moon, P. (2003) *Tohunga Hohepa Kereopa*. David Ling Publishing, Auckland.

Neihardt, J. (1988) *Black Elk speaks: Being the life story of a holy man of the Oglala Sioux*. University of Nebraska Press, Lincoln.

Newman, K. (2009) *Ratana: The prophet*. Penguin, Auckland.

Romme, M., Escher, S., Dillon, J., Corstens, D. & Morris, M. (2009) *Living with voices: 50 stories of recovery*. PCCS Books, Herefordshire.

Sadock, B.J. & Sadock, V.A. (2005) *Kaplan and Sadock's comprehensive textbook of psychiatry* (8th edn). Lippincott Williams & Wilkins, New York.

Somé, M. (1994) *Of water and the spirit*. Putnam, New York.

Tien, A.Y. (1991) 'Distributions of hallucinations in the population'. *Social Psychiatry and Psychiatric Epidemiology* 26: 287–92.

van Os, J., Hanssen, M., Bijl, R.V. & Vollebergh, W. (2001) 'Prevalence of psychotic disorder and community level of psychotic symptoms: An urban-rural comparison'. *Archives of General Psychiatry* 58: 663–68.

8

TĀTAIHONO

Wiremu

This chapter explains what we do when we are working together and how we do it. I would like others to be able to do this mahi (work). I would like to think that Pākehā clinicians and Māori healers, or even indigenous healers and non-indigenous clinicians from other countries, would be able to work together for the benefit of their people. So if there is anything here that is helpful, then kei te pai (this is good).

I liken this way of working to a piece of chewing gum. The basis of a clinician's way of doing things comes from a scientific approach, a medical model. And that's been a good model. Let's say it's like a flash car, like a Ford Falcon V8. Even if you've got the flashest of cars, if one of the spark plugs isn't quite connected properly, if there is a break in the current going into the motor, it will misfire. Then your lovely V8 is only firing on seven cylinders, and it's obvious that something is wrong. But if I'm chewing a piece of gum, I can put that gum onto the broken plug and push it back on, and it will hold it. So now the current can flow evenly again. And even though some people might hesitate to put gum on the engine of their flash car, it can get us where we need to go.

We've taken a simple thing like looking outside the square and applied that. And if you have a reason to think that there might be something cultural going on, then you can ask your healer colleague to join you. This is a very simple intervention, just like the gum. I only need one little piece to hold that plug on. I would liken this to an interruption in the flow of wairua: you push the gum onto the wairua and connect it up again and the flow begins. As far as I'm concerned, when I have a session with someone, the healing power is already there. All I need to do is guide the person to make a spiritual connection by faith to that healing.

Of course, in order to fix your car with the gum, you need to understand how it works. You need to know exactly where to put the gum for it to connect up the flow of electricity again. So there is the understanding and then the practical application. We will address these two parts to our working together: first the principles behind what we do, then the practice.

PRINCIPLES

Wiremu

If you have read the stories in this book, then you will have seen my kōrero about the principles behind what I do. I make a point of explaining these things to whānau. As I said in Chapter 2, 'I hangaia tātou e te kaihanga, kia hīkoi tātou te hīkoi tāngata.' I believe we are first and foremost spiritual beings experiencing a human existence. This principle is the basis for all my mahi.

In the introduction I explained three Māori concepts: mauri, tapu, and mana. You have seen how each of these concepts has come up in our sessions. Helping people gain awareness and understanding is critical so that they can regain authority over their spiritual circumstances. In Chapter 7, Tangi described how learning to act on that understanding made a considerable difference to her sense of well-being. It's not that she stopped having spiritual experiences altogether, but by learning to take charge of her own spiritual space and gradually developing the mana to do that, she was able to regain her well-being.

In terms of understanding why I do what I do, by following our tikanga Māori (customs), I am able to korowai (provide a protective cultural and spiritual cloak for) all of those who are present.

I have an indigenous worldview. What I do comes from my values and beliefs. So in order to be effective in what I do, I hold to those beliefs. We have the belief that we were moulded from the earth, from Papatūānuku, and Te Kaihanga (the creator) breathed into our nostrils and we became living beings. Many other indigenous peoples have a similar belief about coming from the earth, with a deep connection to the land.

Karakia

When we start our session with a karakia, we call it a prayer. However, there is more to it than just a Christian prayer—though it can be that as well. For me, karakia includes giving thanks to the environment, giving thanks to the universe, giving thanks for the fact that we come from our whakapapa, our genealogy, that we have our tīpuna (ancestors), who gave birth to us, who paved the way for us, who sailed the seas, who trod across the land in order that we might exist. Many people lose touch with this sense of themselves and their self-worth because they don't have an answer for a lot of difficulties that are going on for them. In addition to spiritual protection and our connection with Te Kaihanga, karakia serves to whakamana, to enhance the mana of the whānau we are meeting with.

Mihi

When I mihi to the whānau, when I greet them formally according to our tikanga (customs), this also serves to enhance their mana. I'm acknowledging where they are from; I'm acknowledging their environment, their mountains, and their rivers that sustain them. I'm acknowledging that we all have our own heritage, and I'm saying that I'm no better than they are. In order to build rapport, I need to ensure that this is a level playing field. And so by acknowledging their whakapapa and who they are, and by making it clear that I treasure their ancestors and that I will respect whatever their beliefs are, I'm acknowledging their mana.

Taking care of mana is about tiakitanga, guardianship. It's about looking after people and their values and beliefs, treasuring those things, and ensuring that those principles are held in place. Manaakitanga is about being hospitable, embracing a person spiritually or metaphorically. That applies no matter what culture the family comes from. So when we are meeting with families, all the tikanga we use is there to encourage them, to show respect for who they are and where they come from.

Taking care of this is particularly important when we meet whānau who are coming to a mental health service, perhaps for the first time. When we whakamana people, we give them a voice. We give them a voice to have a say in how they think we should be doing things. For example, when an old koroua (male elder) with a rākau (ceremonial staff) gets up to speak on a marae, he holds authority. Nobody will interrupt or speak as long as he has that rākau. When you enter an institution such as a psychiatric unit or a hospital, that rākau is taken away from you; your authority is removed. Our job is to put that rākau back in the hands of the person and the whānau that we are working with.

And so these principles are the ones we hold fast to in the mahi that we are doing together. They are the basis of our working relationship. In Chapter 1 I talked about Tātaihono, which is a spiritual binding together that gives us unity and strength in our partnership. This is important because, although we may not talk about it all the time, we don't forget about the history between our cultures. As I said in Chapter 1, because of that history of colonisation we have to find a way to reconcile and forgive those things that have taken place between our cultures. In addition to that, we come from different points of view. That is a strength of our partnership, but it wouldn't work without manaakitanga. Giving mana to each other is the basis of our mutual respect. Now it's Allister's turn.

Allister

My first comment relates to Wiremu's chewing-gum analogy. It is characteristic of his style that he would humorously downplay his role with such a metaphor. Yet although Wiremu might appear to be minimising the sophistication and subtlety of his healing practice, I think he may be more interested in the underlying message about the nature of wairua as he sees it. In his view, the therapist doesn't have to provide the wairua or electrical current, but the art of healing is in knowing how to reconnect the circuit so that the wairua can flow again.

Wiremu's analogy reminds me of a story told by family therapist Virginia Satir (Satir & Baldwin, 1983). A boilermaker is hired to fix the malfunctioning boiler system of a huge steamship, and after surveying the complicated boiler system thoughtfully, he pulls a small hammer out of the pocket of his overalls and taps a bright-red valve once: this immediately fixes the problem. Satir's point is that the boilermaker's expertise is not so much explained by the impressive nature of his tools and techniques, but by the skill and wisdom of knowing how to use such simple methods. And the most compelling thing for me about Wiremu's work has been the results, which you can see from the stories in this book.

Taking Care of Mana

It will be evident from Wiremu's description in this chapter, as well as the stories of his healing work, that a key part of his focus is on enhancing the mana of those he meets with. Enhancing mana may be a good thing psychologically, but Wiremu is even more interested in the spiritual effect. He views strengthening mana as a very important aspect of spiritual protection for all families.

Although he brings his own considerable mana to the room when meeting with a family and is prepared to use this spiritual authority in the service of the whānau, Wiremu frequently uses humour and other means to make light of his own role, and I notice how this puts families at ease. This works well for him in building a strong bond with the whānau, but even more important from Wiremu's viewpoint is the spiritual protection that is afforded by maintaining his humility. And so Wiremu will whakamana others and whakaiti or 'be the least' himself. And it seems from my Pākehā viewpoint that these aspects might be 'two sides of the same coin' in his healing practice.

Wiremu's concept of manaakitanga can help us draw together themes from the contextual overview in Chapter 2 so that we can find ways of making practical use of those notions in this kind of working partnership. However, before I move onto that, I need to attend to a matter of positioning.

Positioning

I work as a nonindigenous psychiatrist in an indigenous mental health service, which is complicated from a political point of view. Some Māori would take the view that a kaupapa Māori service ought to be 'by Māori, for Māori'. Ideally, from this viewpoint, there may not be a need for Pākehā clinicians in such a Māori service. I have some sympathy for this view, and I see it as part of my role to foster the development of Māori clinicians, including Māori trainee psychiatrists who could fill my role in the future.

Although I have been fortunate to have this opportunity to work at Te Whare Mārie for the last 10 years, I don't consider myself to be an expert on Māori matters or indigenous mental health. We can turn to Wiremu and the writings of psychiatrist colleagues such as Mason Durie (1998, 2009) to assist us in that regard.

There is a range of possible disadvantages to having a Pākehā psychiatrist working in a Māori service. For example, I may be blind to Pākehā discourses that continue to have a subtle—or not so subtle—undermining effect on the development of Māori knowledge and services in mental health. As well as power dynamics implicit in Māori–Pākehā relationships because of the history between our cultures, there are power dynamics that relate to the historical position of doctors in institutions such as ours. I could easily silence indigenous viewpoints inadvertently by the authority I might wield in our team. Perhaps this is one reason why it took me so long to notice what Wiremu had to offer early on.

Fortunately, I have been blessed with forgiving Māori colleagues who have sometimes chosen to challenge me about these matters, either directly or discreetly at a later time. Invariably their courage in doing so has allowed me to learn something about myself. I wonder if this is one aspect of the 'radical compassion' that Linda Tuhiwai Smith (2012) referred to in her quote in Chapter 2.

Alongside that, my command of te reo Māori is poor. With the education and support of Wiremu and our kaumātua at Te Whare Mārie, I can usually get by in formal settings and open a whānau meeting with karakia if required. However, my conversational te reo is very limited. In these ways I am a slower learner than most colleagues at Te Whare Mārie.

I hope it will be apparent that having access to a Māori child and adolescent psychiatrist could be an advantage to Māori whānau and Māori CAF services, and it is my hope that more Māori psychiatrists will be trained and appointed to such services.

Notwithstanding these matters, I am mindful of the privilege—and I also enjoy my role as a child and adolescent psychiatrist. I feel quietly confident that having access to professional expertise in child and adolescent mental health can be useful for Māori families in distress.

So, as a Pākehā clinician in a Māori indigenous setting, what steps can I take to reduce the risk of the inadvertent colonising processes that were outlined in detail in Chapter 2?

Decolonising Approaches and Restoring Mana

If we accept Linda Tuhiwai Smith's (2012) view that 'the whole process of colonization can be viewed as a stripping away of mana', then following Wiremu's example and working to enhance the mana of Māori colleagues and Māori families we are meeting with is a good place to start. For example, it is easy for 'talk space', in the context of a busy professional team meeting, to follow a Pākehā format and be dominated by Western psychological talk. A 'Pākehā decolonising approach' would support kaumātua, the Māori consumer consultant,[1] and Māori clinician colleagues in ensuring that there is Māori tikanga and space for indigenous knowledge to be considered alongside the more dominating clinical paradigms. Of course, finding a good balance isn't easy, and our Māori CAF team has had many conversations about this process over the years.

With Māori families and young people, practices that enhance their sense of self-determination, restore dignity, and affirm their Māori identity are likely to strengthen their mana. I have learnt most about such practices from observing Māori colleagues who do this much more elegantly than I could. An example is Wiremu's interaction with Tangi regarding her experience of her home marae and her Koro at the beginning of Wiremu's first session with her in Chapter 7. Other decolonising practices may include attention to aspects of tikanga or Māori protocol, if the whānau would like this. If we refer to principles in the Treaty of Waitangi, then taking care to foster the partnership with the family we are meeting with and creating a context that encourages their active participation and focuses on their goals and purposes can support the uplifting of their mana.

If colonisation over the last centuries has led to individualistic and secular ways of thinking being foisted on indigenous communities and individuals, then—as Taimalieutu Kiwi Tamasese (2012) described in Chapter 2—unthinking adoption of secular and individual-based therapeutic paradigms could easily perpetuate that same colonisation process. A decolonising focus, therefore, would do well to attend to spiritual matters that are relevant to the indigenous whānau we are meeting with and to honour collective practices inherent in tikanga and the lives of families with whom we come into contact.

At the same time, it behoves us to think critically about the relevance of therapeutic paradigms that we have inherited from the West, that encourage all our focus to be internal to the person. For example, in cognitive behavioural therapy there is a strong focus on the thoughts of the individual client. Psychodynamic therapies focus on a person's internal psychological and emotional processes. Although such practices may be helpful for some young people, we also need to actively promote indigenous therapeutic approaches that connect young people and families to each other, to their places of belonging, to their spirituality, and to their cultures of origin.

One of the striking disruptions caused by colonisation, however, is that many indigenous young people feel cut off from their language, culture, and extended family. If we sincerely want to reverse historical effects of colonisation in our therapeutic work with indigenous young people and families, then we need approaches that promote indigenous identity and ways of being. Te Tuakiri o te Ora is one such Māori therapeutic paradigm (see Chapter 7), another is the Māori relational therapy known as Paiheretia (relational therapy) (Durie, 2003), and a third is the Mahi a Atua therapeutic approach developed by Diana Rangihuna and Lisa Cherrington (Cherrington, 2002). 'Just Therapy' is a family therapy practice that takes account of Māori and Samoan indigenous worldviews (Waldegrave et al., 2003). A further example derived from Pacific indigenous ways of understanding experience is Mana Moana (Mila, 2014): Karlo Mila and her colleague Evangelene Daniela have developed this elegant therapeutic approach into a group programme for Pacific young people called 'The Journey to Motutapu'.

Of course, Māori and other indigenous communities are entitled not only to have access to therapeutic approaches that promote their indigenous identity and worldview, but also to be assured that these approaches work well. Therefore, we have a moral imperative to advocate for resources for indigenous research initiatives and collaborations that can contribute to an evidence base of effective indigenous therapeutic practices.

Mitzi Nairn (2002), a Pākehā Treaty educator, has suggested that 'the descendants of the colonisers have different decolonisation tasks from the descendants of the colonised'. For Pākehā clinicians, it is our responsibility to learn to recognise varieties of anti-Māori discourse, such as those identified by Tim McCreanor (2012) and Ray Nairn (see Chapter 2), and to use our professional influence to challenge these taken-for-granted Pākehā ways of talking and thinking about Māori.

The best way that I know for developing 'discursive resources' to expand our repertoire of 'decolonising discourses' is by listening carefully to Māori colleagues and kaumātua, giving their explanations for the predicaments of families we may be meeting with. If they know something of the whakapapa or genealogy of a particular family, often they are able to shed some historical light on the background of this family some generations before. I find this helps me step back from my immediate judgements about families immersed in multiple types of adversity. That way I try to refrain from individualising the problems they face, such as poverty, drug use, and gang affiliations. And the next step is finding ways to articulate these resources so that they are more available to other team members and Pākehā colleagues.

Pākehā Views on Māori–Pākehā Partnerships

Pākehā education researcher Alex Barnes has gathered advice from the experience of Pākehā education researchers who have endeavoured to take a decolonising approach to 'the Māori–Pākehā hyphen' (Barnes, 2013). Participants spoke of the need to respond to relationships with 'heart, care [and] respect', and of the benefits of 'leaving your ego at the door'. They talked of the need for 'careful listening' and the importance of developing an awareness of when Pākehā knowledge becomes overbearing and ceases to be useful for the Māori collective. Mindful of the need to be cognisant of power relationships, they pointed out that choosing an 'unknowing position' can be unsettling for some Pākehā, but may provide for a much more valuable learning opportunity. They emphasised that the values of reciprocity in Māori culture mean that, for those Pākehā who have been given access to Māori knowledge or learning, there is an implicit obligation to give something back, and this may well mean a 'commitment to build and sustain relationships over a long period'. Other authors have noted that such obligations may extend to the need to take political action. This may be uncomfortable territory for some clinicians. The Royal Australian and New Zealand College of Psychiatrists' guidelines for Aboriginal and Torres Strait Islander mental health highlight the political implications of indigenous health interventions: they point out that working in this area may necessitate questioning government policy and challenging community attitudes that are negatively affecting the well-being of indigenous peoples (Durie et al., 2009).

Applying Principles of Cultural Accountability

One important way to address the historical and current relationships between indigenous and settler practitioners is to attend to processes and practices of cultural accountability. Collective practices that facilitate this in institutions or agencies were described from the work of the Just Therapy team in Chapter 1.

When Wiremu and I are meeting with a family, we are accountable to the family for the work that we do in partnership with them. We are also accountable to their culture of origin, and, of course, any such family may have different tribal affiliations than Wiremu and may vary considerably in the extent to which they have retained these links.

On another level, Wiremu considers that he is accountable to the wairua, or spiritual realm.

In matters of Māori culture, as a Pākehā psychiatrist I consider myself accountable to Wiremu. Consequently, on all matters of tikanga, or Māori protocols or Māori knowledge, I defer to Wiremu's expert opinion. I would regard his view as the final word on such matters.

Finally, in our indigenous service, cultural accountability processes in our multidisciplinary team meetings mean that we would defer to the views of the elders, or kaumātua, present on matters of tikanga, or Māori culture, just as we would to the consumer consultant on our team for matters relating to the experience of whaiora or clients.

Safety First

In our work together we have to attend to other lines of clinical accountability as well as other legal forms of accountability, such as those pertaining to child protection. Sometimes finding the right balance can take quite some time for discussion and consideration. A frequent dilemma in the context of mental health services relates to considerations of risk and safety of those we are meeting with and those around them: this matter comes up in Tangi's story on several occasions.

In general, Wiremu and I have taken the joint position that can be summarised as 'safety first'. For example, if a young person is hearing a voice telling them to kill themselves or someone else and there is a dilemma about whether the voice they are hearing is an auditory hallucination indicating a form of psychotic illness or a cultural experience indicating a spiritual problem, we would resort to the 'safety first' principle. This might involve arranging for the young person to be contained in a safer environment such as a hospital facility to allow further assessment of both the psychiatric and cultural aspects of their presentation.

PRACTICE

Wiremu

This collaboration that I call Tātaihono requires commitment and effort from both sides. Being able to have open and honest kōrero together helps us sort out any misunderstandings that can easily crop up between our Māori and Pākehā viewpoints. When Allister and I work together, quite a bit of the mahi has already been done before I get to meet with the whānau. For readers who are health professionals, I encourage you to read what Allister has to say about this.

Allister

Before talking further about our way of working together, we acknowledge the context of our collaboration. Wiremu and I met and worked together at Te Whare Mārie. As we described in Chapter 1, in this indigenous context we are expected to give primacy to Māori worldviews alongside our clinical worldviews. Our kaumātua (elders), Māori consumer consultant, and fellow kaimahi (clinicians) encourage us to consider cultural interpretations of people's symptoms and experiences alongside clinical concerns.

Steps in Identifying Cultural and Spiritual Problems

From time to time a young person will be referred to us with a problem that appears distinctly cultural in nature. An example of that is Caleb's story (see Chapter 5): the vivid visual description he gave of seeing a Māori warrior convinced his Māori clinician at the Early Intervention Service that he could be suffering from a cultural problem, and they referred him on to Te Whare Mārie for further assessment.

Sometimes a clinician at our service will suspect a cultural problem from the information provided on a written referral to our service. But most commonly such matters arise during our first meeting with a family or at a later meeting.

Pathways of Enquiry

When I first meet with a young person and their family, I listen for any experiences they relate that indicate that cultural and spiritual experiences are familiar to them. Alternatively, such experiences may be confusing or distressing for the young person. Various pathways in the interview might open up a conversation about these territories of experience.

Listening to the Detail

One pathway is by listening to the detail of their experience of the problem. In George's situation, he was suffering from nonepileptic seizures and hearing a voice that reduced somewhat with a low dose of antipsychotic medicine. I was wondering about psychosis as an explanation—and I could have asked George questions that would narrow down the conversation and make it less likely that any alternative explanation could emerge. Standard psychiatric interviewing questions can take the form of closed questions: 'Is the voice internal or external to your head? Are there any commands to harm yourself or someone else? Is the voice providing a running commentary?'

However, when I listened to George's description, the more detail I heard, the more it sounded like something other than psychosis. He talked about a 'thing' hanging around near him, and he described its colour. This enquiry required an open style of question: 'What was this experience like for you? Please describe the experience in as much detail as you can.' In response, George described something that didn't quite fit into my paradigm: 'It feels like I've got this 24-hour-a-day bully. It feels like I've got this thing behind my right shoulder.'

When young people like George and Tangi provide such vivid descriptions and Wiremu then confirms some of their experiences with his own descriptions of the same entities, it has been possible to map their descriptions to his understanding of the terrain in this territory of experience. I have noticed some cultural patterns emerging in their descriptions, and my future enquiries with other families are informed by the experiences shared by these young people. If a young person's detailed description reminds me of other cultural descriptions I've heard, then I would consider whether they may be experiencing something spiritual or cultural.

George described the 'thing' that was impinging on him as located in space. He could identify particular qualities it had as if he was perceiving it with a range of senses, including visual (colour), auditory (voice), and feeling ('feels bad'). Andrew Sims (1995) reports in his textbook *Symptoms in the Mind* a case of visual and auditory hallucinations occurring synchronously in a person with temporal lobe epilepsy; but apart from that I have only rarely come across references to such detailed descriptions of synchronous or well-integrated 'hallucinations' in psychiatric writing. However, Wiremu commonly describes spiritual experiences in which he can see a figure talking and hear the words they appear to be saying at the same time.

Experiences in the Whānau

When other family members have had similar spiritual or cultural experiences or know about them, this can be another fruitful pathway of enquiry. I often ask about such matters before enquiring about mental health problems in the family, as most Māori and Pacific families assume that psychiatrists interpret unusual experiences as signs of madness. I might introduce this idea by saying: 'Many Māori and Pacific families view spiritual experiences as normal. For example, some people have a strong feeling that a deceased family member is still around. Does anyone in your family have experiences like that?' If families are adamant that these kinds of experiences are not part of their lives, I would leave that topic and move on. If they seem unsure but curious and perhaps sceptical about my sincerity, I might suggest another example: 'In some families certain people have dreams that come true and this is viewed as a kind of spiritual experience.' Or else: 'In other families, someone may feel a ghostly presence in a room at home. Maybe it feels good or bad to them.' Other examples relate to places:

> 'Some people visit certain places and notice a distinct good or bad feeling about the place. They can't explain it, but they are quite sure about it. From a Western point of view this might be hard to explain, but for Māori or Pacific families these experiences might be considered spiritual. How do you view these kinds of happenings?'

Many Māori whānau have family members—often an elder—who are very familiar with spiritual experiences and comfortable talking about them. Recently I met a mother who had brought her son to our service because she was concerned about the possibility of depression. When I asked if she considered there could be a spiritual problem contributing to this, she said, 'I know what you're talking about. I've had a lot of those kind of experiences. I'm quite confident this is not a spiritual problem. If it was I'd know about it.' She spoke with considerable authority, dismissing this as a 'spiritual problem'. I expect that if I had suggested a consultation with Wiremu, she might have replied, 'I'm sure I would get on well with Wiremu, but I don't think my son has a mate Māori problem.'

In other situations, the family believes there is a spiritual problem and I'm interested to understand how they came to that conclusion. Moana's story in Chapter 6 illustrates this very well. Moana's mother Tere came to see us and said at the outset, 'I think my daughter has a cultural problem, I think she may be possessed.' And because of her convictions, I was curious about her reasons. When I learnt about her background, I realised she had considerable spiritual and cultural knowledge and understanding and was genuinely grappling with and confused about what was going on with her daughter: I needed to hear Tere's account in its entirety before I could reach a conclusion. While I was still considering explanations such as dissociation and possible trauma, I was thinking, 'Is there a way to address this problem from the point of view of the family's culture of origin?'

Consequently, in talking with whānau, I hope to create space for us to jointly consider two contrasting but overlapping domains: the spiritual or cultural domain, and the psychiatric or psychological domain. And I want them to understand that I'm open to the validity of both perspectives. But more than this, in an indigenous service, this is a legitimate conversation for us to be having. And I might say, 'If your whānau are not into this, that's absolutely fine.' Most families are resolute about this. They may say, 'We don't believe in that stuff, it's not relevant for us, but thank you for asking.' Or, by contrast, they might be adamant: 'I know exactly what you are talking about.' This latter response is far more frequent. They may go on to share their reminiscences—for example, they may talk about an aunty whom they go to in the whānau to address wairua matters. Or someone might say, 'I've never had any spiritual experiences myself . . . although there was that one time after Uncle died that I had this funny feeling . . . but that's the only time.' This context of respectful reminiscence may trigger another story, and before long there may be several similar narratives. Even after a brief conversation like this, it becomes far easier to communicate about this territory of their experiences, if necessary, later on.

Enquiring about Early Experiences

Another pathway is the history of this kind of awareness in the young person's life. From a child psychiatrist's point of view, this parallels what we call a developmental history. But here we are focusing on 'spirituality' in the broadest sense. I might ask, 'Were there any times when you thought that your child was having some kind of spiritual experience when they were little?' Parents or grandparents might respond, 'No, nothing like that.' Or they might recall one example, which often leads to two or three other stories—and suddenly this young person's history reveals a track record of experiences of this kind. My Māori colleagues refer to such young people as spiritually 'tuned in'. With this whakapapa, whānau, and developmental background in a young person troubled by odd perceptual experiences, it's a valid question to ask if these experiences could be spiritual.

We have highlighted three pathways for approaching cultural and spiritual territories of experience. The first is listening for the detail of the young person's experience and noticing distinctions that don't quite fit with psychosis or other psychiatric paradigms. The second is asking about other family members with previous spiritual experiences. And the third entails an enquiry into whether the young person has a history of such experiences in their past.

Diagnostic Distinctions

Another pathway I use for approaching spiritual and cultural experiences is to think carefully about a possible diagnosis. As a psychiatrist, it is part of my training to look carefully at the pattern of distress that a person is describing in their lives to see if this fits with other well-described patterns, which we call diagnostic categories. Identifying a known pattern can point us toward a well-tried and tested solution for that problem. However, many people both within and outside psychiatry have criticised the modern preoccupation with expanding diagnostic categories (such as some of those outlined in the recently launched *Diagnostic and Statistical Manual of Mental Disorders* [DSM-5] (American Psychiatric Association, 2013)) to cover many more areas of human experience (Watters, 2010). These critics say that such categories go too far in 'medicalising' human distress.

Although I acknowledge these concerns, I have seen many situations in which a diagnostic label has given a person and their family power to take action against the problem and has assisted them in freeing themselves from its grip. If we are looking at mapping out what might or might not be cultural and spiritual territories of experience, then diagnostic categories can also offer useful guidance. For example, if a young person talks about hearing a voice, they are frequently fearful that their experience indicates a serious mental illness. In George's situation in Chapter 4, when he spoke initially about hearing a voice, he was immediately referred to EIS, who work with young people during their first episode of a serious psychotic illness. Tangi, in Chapter 7, had been hearing voices and having other experiences for some years, but didn't reveal them to us for more than 18 months because she was afraid we would think she was 'mental' and that she might have schizophrenia.

In psychiatry there is an ongoing debate about the nature of schizophrenia; some experts believe it will turn out to be a group of related or unrelated conditions (Sadock & Sadock, 2005). In spite of intense research, the diagnostic criteria have remained relatively unchanged over the last 20 years. A young person who is hearing a voice or voices, and even seeing apparitions or other visions as well, may still not meet the criteria that would qualify for a diagnosis of schizophrenia. Even if the voices or visions are classified as hallucinations, the criteria for this condition require other symptoms of a psychotic illness, such as severely disorganised thinking or behaviour, or delusions[2] or 'negative symptoms'.[3] Even when Tangi was feeling most tormented by her experiences, she was not showing signs of delusions, disorganised thinking or behaviour, or negative symptoms. Accordingly, if we follow the DSM diagnostic classification carefully, she could not be diagnosed with schizophrenia. This distinction gives us diagnostic grounds to step back from that label and consult with a cultural expert such as a Māori healer to allow consideration of a cultural context or spiritual cause for the problem. Despite the biomedical emphasis in modern psychiatry, even the DSM classification advocates for cultural and spiritual factors to be considered as part of an overall understanding of a person's predicament (American Psychiatric Association, 2013). For example, so-called false beliefs would not be considered delusions if they are consistent with the cultural background of the person or the religious beliefs of others in their community.

Diagnosis and Age

An additional distinction can be made about the age of onset of a problem. Studies indicate that symptoms of major psychotic illnesses commonly emerge in people between their late teenage years and early thirties (Sadock & Sadock, 2005). Such problems are considered rare before puberty, and hardly ever occur in preschoolers. So when Moana, at the age of 10, reported seeing an old lady in the corner of her bedroom and hearing a voice, she was in an age group where psychosis is less likely and other possible explanations ought to be considered. Tangi's description of hearing a voice before she was nine would be considered unusually young for the first onset of a psychotic illness. On the other hand, Tangi and George described hearing, seeing, and feeling things that they considered to be spiritual over many years, going back to their early primary school years at least. Wiremu recalls his first spiritual experiences at the age of three. On this basis, when a young person talks about unexplained perceptual experiences at an early age, alongside other explanations (such as possible traumatic reexperiencing, or even a medical condition such as epilepsy) I would consider whether or not the young person might be spiritually aware and would then consider offering the family a consultation with Wiremu, if they would welcome that.

Holding Different Possibilities in Mind

One challenge is having the confidence, as a psychiatrist or mental health clinician, not to jump to conclusions about diagnoses and causes. We sometimes need to mentally juggle several paradigms and defer reaching a final conclusion pending further cultural and clinical assessment, exploration, and understanding. What is confronting the young person, their whānau, and me may turn out to be a 'blend' of cultural and clinical problems that needs to be considered biculturally so as not to compromise one version at the expense of another.

Tangi's story (see Chapter 7) provides a good example of this. Her sudden revelation about hearing a voice and the dramatic change in her demeanour two weeks after she first met Wiremu forced us to reconsider our previous understanding of her problems, our formulation, and possible diagnoses. In my mind I was concerned she was developing a serious psychotic illness, but I knew we needed to continue to consider several possible explanations. Accordingly, I said to Tangi, 'I can think of three possible explanations right now for that voice that you are experiencing.' Drawing on the whiteboard, I explained that her voice could be a psychotic experience, or a result of past trauma, or it might still be a spiritual problem. I reminded her that Wiremu had met with her and previously confirmed that some of her experiences seemed to have a spiritual origin. There were other possibilities, such as a medical problem causing the voices, but those were the three options I considered most likely.

While we waited for the next opportunity to consult with Wiremu, Tangi commenced antipsychotic medication, but we agreed that we were still holding three possibilities in mind and not foreclosing on spiritual factors playing a part in her distress. We did not rule out psychosis, because her experience was consistent with a psychotic problem; in fact, Tangi believed that her voice was a psychotic experience. However, at our subsequent meeting with Wiremu, he concluded that her voice originated from a spiritual problem and, after his intervention, the voice disappeared.

Nine months after this incident, during Tangi's further period of crisis, we were able to take action to address her safety without having to draw a final conclusion about the primary cause of her problem—whether it was psychosis, trauma, or spiritual. We could continue to hold each possibility in mind and work closely with our colleagues on the adolescent unit to share our understanding of her problem.

Holding several alternative explanations in mind allows us to travel along the borders of these two worlds and crisscross between them as required by the demands of the situation. At each point it is vital that the young person and their family are engaged in the negotiation about how to proceed, at a pace that works for them.

Presenting a Formulation Back to the Family

At Te Whare Mārie, Te Pounamu[4] is a common method that we use to facilitate the development of a shared understanding of the overall problem and situation with whānau (Ruha, 2007). Towards the end of our first meeting, I often put up a diagram on the whiteboard that links together key matters that I've heard from the young person and their whānau. Once it's on the board, I summarise the story the family have told me, emphasising the dynamic interplay between different aspects. I request their response and we amend the diagram based on their suggestions. This shared understanding of the overall situation allows us to then develop a shared plan of action.

Talking to the Team

As soon as practicable after the initial family meeting, I talk to our Māori CAFS multidisciplinary team, outlining the detail of the assessment so far, drawing up the shared Te Pounamu formulation, and explaining the family's priorities and goals. Our team, which includes kaumātua, a Māori consumer consultant, and clinicians including social workers, nurses, and psychologists, has a culture of talking openly about wairua matters alongside all the other psychological, relational, and physical health aspects, and it has maintained this culture after Wiremu's departure. Since he left the team and returned to the Gisborne area, for some years Wiremu continued to visit our service from time to time and was able to offer consultations for Māori CAFS clients. From that time, a referral to Wiremu required the agreement of the kaumātua and the multidisciplinary team, and the team would also suggest other options. These included offering the whānau the opportunity to see the kaumātua first or referral to other healers in the local community with whom the whānau might have connections.

Of course, finding or replacing someone like Wiremu may be very difficult. There are many barriers to Māori healers being employed alongside mental health clinicians in state-funded health care services. These services generally don't have policies and procedures in place that facilitate the employment of Māori healers. The requirement for university qualifications would exclude many tohunga. Even if a specific position was created, attracting a Māori healer with the requisite gift and skill, as well as a willingness to work in a government-funded mental health service alongside clinicians who may have little knowledge of what they can offer, may not be easy.

Detailed accounts of Wiremu's sessions with families can be found in several chapters, including those pertaining to George (Chapter 4), Moana (Chapter 6), and Tangi (Chapter 7).

Making Distinctions

Forming a conclusion about what is going on when a young person presents with unusual experiences is a considerable dilemma for me as a psychiatrist. If we accept that a young person could have a spiritual problem but it looks like a psychiatric problem such as psychosis, how can we reliably make a distinction between the two? It's much easier to take the perspective that all of these experiences are psychiatric in origin. There are no roadmaps in psychiatry to help us distinguish between psychiatric problems and spiritual experiences. Wiremu does not say that everything is a spiritual problem. He does maintain that wairua is relevant to everyone's situation, and often aspects of that can be addressed. However some of Wiremu's most helpful advice has been when he has concluded that a young person doesn't have a spiritual problem. Let me describe a few examples.

Wiremu was asked to see Aroha, a 17-year-old Māori woman who had been admitted to the rangatahi unit (adolescent psychiatry unit). Aroha had been hearing voices and said that she had seen her deceased father. Her thoughts seemed muddled. At times she seemed suspicious of staff and had very little to say. The team was concerned about the severity of her illness, but at the same time her family and some team members wondered if she might have a cultural problem. Aroha came from the same iwi area as Wiremu, and he was familiar with some of her extended family members. After two meetings with her, Wiremu's assessment was that he could not detect a mate Māori problem or other spiritual cause for her experiences. Wiremu's finding reassured the family and allowed the team to proceed more confidently with treatment for her psychotic illness.

We asked Wiremu to see Stan, a 14-year-old Māori boy who was in a Māori residential programme because of running away, robberies, and problems in previous care and protection placements. Earlier, Stan had described seeing his deceased grandfather, whom he had been very close to, on the end of his bed at night. Recently Stan had threatened a staff member with a knife in the kitchen of his residence: he said that a voice had told him to stab someone, and that had happened several times. He did not appear to have other psychotic symptoms, and the programme managed this threatening behaviour in a matter-of-fact way with appropriate behavioural consequences. When Wiremu met with him, he quickly drew the conclusion that Stan had fabricated the story about hearing a voice: he didn't think there was a spiritual problem or a psychotic one. When he raised this, Stan admitted he had made it up.

On another occasion, Wiremu was asked to see Kevin, an 18-year-old Māori man who had been referred a month before by his family doctor. The doctor was concerned he might be depressed and had already started him on antidepressant medication. At that time Kevin said that he had been hearing his deceased Pākehā grandmother's voice talking to him. We agreed on a plan to assist him, and I raised the matter about his grandmother with Wiremu in a multidisciplinary team meeting two weeks later. Straight after the meeting, Wiremu mentioned that during that discussion, he had seen a woman in the room who he surmised had appeared there because she was connected to Kevin. Judging from her appearance, he was confident that she was Māori.

Within a couple of weeks Kevin's situation worsened. He appeared very distressed and had been hiding in a cupboard at home. He had stopped caring for himself. On the day he was seen, he had walked into the middle of the road amid oncoming traffic, and he was only partly clothed despite the wintry conditions. Bystanders were concerned and the police had been called. Wiremu was invited to join the acute assessment that day. His conclusion was that the young man was definitely unwell and needed to be in a hospital. Wiremu didn't think that a spiritual problem could account for Kevin's predicament, and he said that he had not detected anything that would lead him to think that Kevin's Pākehā grandmother was spiritually present or influencing the situation. He wondered if the woman he had seen in the meeting two weeks before might be a Māori ancestor of Kevin's, but on the basis of his perception of the young man's wairua, as well as his descriptions of the voices and his grandmother, Wiremu deduced that she was not likely to be the source of the voices. Wiremu strongly supported his colleague's view that urgent inpatient admission for further assessment and treatment was required.

For someone who is not familiar with Wiremu's work, these findings might seem to be hard to fathom. Of course, from a Western scientific point of view, it would be impossible to verify his conclusions. Nevertheless, when these case stories are placed alongside the stories included elsewhere in this book, it becomes apparent that Wiremu's cultural and spiritual assessment findings are quite specific to the circumstances of each young person and their whānau. In each of these cases his conclusions contributed to key decisions about appropriate ways to assist the young person and were a guide to clinicians attempting to include cultural and spiritual factors in their overall assessment and formulation. Wiremu's determination that spiritual factors are not likely to be the main problem can be just as helpful as times when he concludes that they are.

Wiremu

In my mahi I often use a process of elimination so that I am working through different possible causes of 'spiritual dis-ease' and using various spiritual clues to confirm or eliminate my spiritual hypotheses. For me, it is valuable in this collaboration to have the clinical backup, so that if something doesn't appear to be mainly a spiritual problem, I can turn to Allister for his expertise. I think it is crucial not only to have an understanding of the spiritual side, but also to have an understanding of the mental side. I am always asking if a fellow healer who is working within a mental health service or clinic has the training to recognise if a person is actually psychotic. I think it is really important that we don't discard the possibility that someone is having some brain problem that causes them to lose touch with reality. It is important that healers are aware that there can be such things as a physical problem in the brain or something that is not functioning properly because of a deficiency. Drugs and alcohol, for example, can cause such an imbalance: attending to the spiritual side could still help that person, but they may well need treatment to help with the physical problem as well.

Allister

Distinguishing Psychosis from Spiritual Experiences

What can we conclude, as psychiatrists and other mental health professionals, about how to distinguish psychotic and spiritual experiences when we are faced with trying to assist an indigenous person who is having unusual and disturbing experiences?

For us this is a work in progress, and there are many other colleagues who could more eloquently contribute to this project of putting language to these distinctions in mental health. As with Wiremu's chewing-gum analogy, we could try turning to a complicated system of analysis such as the Ford Falcon V8, or we could focus on simple principles like the gum.

For me, the principles may be the most helpful. Listening to the details of the person's experience and carrying out a careful psychiatric assessment is nothing more than good psychiatry. Asking about early spiritual experiences as part of a developmental history and enquiring about family members who may have had spiritual experiences can easily be included in questions about family history. Perhaps there are some patterns that might alert us to the possibility of a spiritual component to what is going on. For example, it may be that seeing and hearing a deceased relative talking to you is more likely to be spiritual than psychotic. What about an experience in which the auditory and visual elements are in synchrony? In other situations, it makes sense that some experiences that are culturally or personally meaningful for the person and their family may be more likely to be cultural or spiritual in origin.

As outlined earlier, careful consideration of diagnostic detail is another aspect of everyday psychiatric practice that can alert me to possible spiritual concerns. So-called auditory hallucinations in the absence of other symptoms of a severe psychotic disorder, such as disorganised thinking or delusional beliefs, may be reasonable grounds for considering a consultation with an indigenous healer colleague. On the other hand, if we accept that people can have spiritual experiences, then people experiencing psychosis may be just as likely to have spiritual experiences in their lives, even alongside their psychotic experiences. So 'either/or' thinking may not serve us well in all cases. But as we have seen in these stories, sometimes it can be very helpful for a young person and their family if a distinction can be made.

However, focusing on too much analysis of the form and content of the experiences may ultimately be fruitless. All I need to do as a psychiatrist is be able to recognise some indicators that alert me to a possible spiritual component and the need to consult with Wiremu. In this spiritual sphere, where I am out of the scope of my training and expertise, I will always have to rely on my indigenous colleague who has the spiritual and cultural expertise to help us all discern the spiritual and cultural elements of the young person's situation. Indigenous healers of the calibre of Wiremu are in short supply, so we will need to be discerning about which young people in our mental health service could most benefit from Wiremu's kind of expertise.

Perhaps the most important principle is the 'gum' that makes up the Tātaihono partnership. Of course, I could just suggest to the family that they consult an indigenous healer known to them in their community, and perhaps they could relay to me the results of that consultation. However, if we are all able to work together, we can develop a shared formulation or map to try to help all of us understand what may be going on. As we have seen in Tangi's story, not all problems are amenable to quick-fix solutions. Therefore, having a partnership with an indigenous healer colleague and the person and their family that allows the ongoing development of this kind of shared understanding can allow us to continue working together closely over time through the difficult terrain of human distress. It can allow us to attend to both the indigenous viewpoints of the family and healer and the psychiatry viewpoints. It can assist us in reviewing together the outcomes of the family's solutions, the indigenous healing interventions, and psychiatry interventions. And if some matters remain unresolved, such a shared formulation can be a starting point for us to consider together what to do next.

HOW THIS BOOK WAS WRITTEN

Allister

When Wiremu asked me to join him in writing a book about our work together, I had little idea what that would entail. The style of the book was developed in collaboration with David while we were writing an article about Moana's story, which became the basis for Chapter 6. Wiremu's words were audiorecorded over many hours of our conversations about his work, his views, and the young people and families we had met and after joint talks to medical meetings and conference workshops, where we presented a number of these stories with the blessing of the families concerned. From these recordings, I then pieced together his words into text as faithfully as I could and emailed the stories to David. It is through Wiremu's wisdom and humour as a healer and David's skill as an editor that these stories have been brought to life. Moana's story went through more than 20 iterations of this back-and-forth process, as well as returning to Wiremu to check that his words had been accurately rendered and to find out what else he wanted to add. While we were writing Moana's story I showed the manuscript to her mother Tere, and her rich responses meant that it was quickly apparent that her voice was a necessary addition to the story. Again, with her consent, I recorded her words and rendered them into text before returning them to her for her corrections and additions. This same process was used for all the young people and family members who give voice to their views in this book.

TĀTAIHONO AND THE SHARING OF MĀORI KNOWLEDGE

Allister

During the preparation of this chapter, David suggested that the three of us sit down together and have a conversation about the nature of the learning experiences that Wiremu was offering me in our work together over several years. He had noticed over the course of editing each of the chapters certain ways in which Wiremu would help my understanding about wairua. As we talked, David addressed Wiremu:

David: I know you have your own ways of teaching, but it's not reciprocal. You're not wanting to know about psychiatric knowledge in the same way that Allister has had a desire to learn about your viewpoint. Allister is working in a bicultural service, and I suspect he considers that he has a

> moral and ethical responsibility to be more than just a psychiatrist who happens to work in a bicultural agency. After each chapter and over time, it appeared to me that Allister was becoming more and more your apprentice.

My initial response to David's comment was a feeling of discomfort. If apprenticing myself to Wiremu was to in any way suggest that I was aspiring to be a Māori healer, then that didn't fit for me—apart from it being impossible for a range of obvious reasons. In addition, I am satisfied with my role as a psychiatrist and don't feel I need to relinquish that. But I had been keen to understand more about Wiremu's point of view and experiences of wairua, because that seemed important to many of the Māori families I was meeting with. As our conversation unfolded I realised that several key learning moments stood out in my mind, and Wiremu had approached them in particular ways.

In Caleb's story it had not been at all obvious to me how Caleb picking up a piece of pounamu that didn't belong to him could cause his dramatic experience of seeing and hearing the warrior figure outside his gate. Wiremu patiently guided me through the key Māori concepts to help me understand this. He also noted that addressing the problem spiritually had apparently solved it.

In George's story, I was impressed with Wiremu's approach to the initial family session, but I had no expectation that such a simple intervention as Wiremu's karakia would fix this dramatic problem in such a short timeframe. Wiremu made a point of giving me the task of catching up with George to see how he was progressing so that I could see the results for myself.

Later, with Moana, I was nonplussed about Wiremu's description after the session of the different figures that he could see in the room, and I didn't know what to make of that. Again Wiremu asked me to check this observation with the family. It was months later when I heard from Tere that the wider family had been able to exactly identify the figures. For me this was a vivid experience that illustrated graphically what Wiremu talked about when he spoke of matters coming 'down the generations'.

Another example of a moment when I was floored and unable to reconcile what I was being presented with was when Wiremu reported his experience of the silent 'screaming woman' that had occurred 500 kilometres away, but on the same evening when Tangi had reported being tormented by her 'screeching lady'. Because I was the one on the phone to both of them, I had an experience of having to make sense of something that was very challenging to my usual understanding of everyday life. David put it well during our conversation:

David: So do you think there is something in your apprenticeship of Allister, where he has to flounder, he has to fathom something out. You can't just give him a simple answer. He has to find his own way through it and struggle, and quibble with himself to . . .

Wiremu: . . . interpret, or translate. Yes. Doesn't that make for better learning? If you were going to teach me arithmetic, you're not going to sit there and do the sums for me. I have to learn. And I would arrive at my own answers, be they wrong or right. Then you may correct me and say, 'Hang on a minute, if you had taken that and put that there you might get a different answer.'

David: Yeah, but this knowledge is kind of like, embodied, or experiential. You have to experience it. You can't just read a book on it. You have to be there, to be amongst it in order to begin to believe in it. Allister surely has every right to be suspicious.

Wiremu: Of course. I'm always suspicious!

As a psychiatrist, I believe that it is possible for me to work alongside Wiremu as a Māori healer effectively, without necessarily sharing the same belief system that he holds. I don't have to believe that everything he does works and accept it unthinkingly. However, there does need to be basic trust and mutual respect between us. From my point of view, that appeared to develop gradually between us over the two or three years after we began working at Te Whare Mārie. However, when David asked Wiremu about this, he saw it differently.

Wiremu

David: Why did you trust Allister to write this book with you?

Wiremu: Because I was told to. I can't explain it. I was drawn to do that by the wairua. Even before we were actually sitting down and working together, that trust was already there.

When Allister and I were seeing families together, I didn't really think that I was teaching him about wairua. I didn't see it that way. What I *was* doing was sharing and giving him the mana to share that understanding with others. I think I had the same approach that I have with families. As far as I am concerned, the whānau always has the mana. They're in control. They're piloting the plane. I'm just here to move the cargo around and, if they don't like it, I can put on a parachute and jump off the plane. And it's the same with Allister. When we were working together and he would ask me questions, he had the mana. And, of course, at the beginning I would respond to where his understanding about wairua was up to. It was like, 'Let's start off on this level.' Maybe the answers that I gave him then were meant to be simple. They were meant to be instructive. I wanted to be very clear about what I thought was taking place. And if I didn't see anything, I would say that I didn't pick anything up—so that Allister might realise that there are certain times when I *could* pick those things up. And I would encourage him to do the karakia at the beginning of the session so that he would develop the confidence to do that, and after a while it started to flow.

With regard to Caleb, I think that the challenge to Allister's thinking was, 'Is this a psychotic episode or is it a spiritual experience?' After the intervention of the tohunga, Caleb's disturbing experiences stopped. At that point, my role was to assist Allister to make sense of this, step by step. I'd already been told by the wairua to take time to do that.

As for my description of Moana's ancestors, I knew that Allister was curious about that, but I figured we would get there in the end. That's why I put it in his court to ask Tere about what the family made of that. In the case of George, I knew that as a doctor and a psychiatrist, Allister would have to explore and carry out that process of elimination to determine in his mind what might have been going on for George. I also knew that the particular thing that he couldn't see was sitting right there. I wasn't surprised that George improved quickly after our session because I could see her and so was confident in the intervention from my source.

When Allister rang me after speaking with Tangi, I immediately understood that the screaming woman that had passed over me two nights before was related to Tangi. I figured that Allister might be surprised about that. That's why I asked him to check with Tangi about the timing of her experience. Because given that I was so far away, how the heck would I have known that this screaming banshee that passed over me at nine o'clock that night was related to her? Now, seeing as Allister was the one doing the phoning, he was left to try to get his head around that one. But it wasn't me giving him that learning experience. Like I said, it's the wairua. And so one purpose for me in this is to help Allister understand more about a Māori point of view so that he can spot a situation when someone with spiritual experiences might be misdiagnosed.

Allister: So it's like an extra skill for a psychiatrist in a bicultural setting or a Māori setting?

Wiremu: No, it's giving you a gift as a person. You have your own spirituality and your own heart and soul, that gives you that feeling. So, it is about helping you understand as a person first and as a doctor second. I am happy for you to learn as a doctor as well, because then I hope you'll be less likely to misdiagnose anybody. That's always been my thing about making people aware, so that we as Māori won't be misunderstood.

The key for me is understanding. If Allister is able to develop that understanding of wairua and consider that alongside his other knowledge as a psychiatrist, then he is capable of looking outside the box of Western thinking. He'll never be a Māori, but he can be a healer in the broad sense of that word, because having that awareness that a problem could be spiritual may have a healing effect for a young person and their whānau. So you've just added another kete to the kete of knowledge that you follow and know well. And that allows you to deliver the best service that you possibly can. Āpirana Ngata (Ngata, 1993: p. xi) was addressing us as Māori, but his whakatauākī sums up this idea very well:

> E tipu, e rea,
> Mo nga rā o tōu ao;
> Ko to ringa ki nga rākau a te Pākehā
> Hei ara mo to tinana
> Ko to ngākau ki nga taonga a o tīpuna Maori
> Hei tikitiki mo to mahuna,
> A, ko to wairua ki to Atua,
> Nāna nei nga mea katoa.
>
> ('Grow young shoot for the future that is before you. Turn your hand to the technology of the Pākehā to ensure your livelihood. Retain the teachings of your ancestors as a legacy for the generations to come. Give your spirit to God, the creator of all.')

Notes

1. The Māori consumer consultant at Te Whare Mārie is an indigenous mental health service user employed by our service to advocate for the perspectives of Māori service users in the planning and day-to-day running of the service and is a valued participant in multidisciplinary team meetings.
2. A delusion is a false belief based on an incorrect conclusion about external reality that a person remains convinced of despite obvious evidence to the contrary and which is well out of step with what others from their culture or subculture would be likely to accept (see DSM5).
3. Negative symptoms refer to a person suffering from markedly reduced motivation, talking, emotional responsiveness, and enjoyment in their life over an extended period (Sadock & Sadock, 2005).
4. Te Pounamu is a Māori visual formulation tool developed by Peta Ruha and Te Whare Mārie in which different aspects of the young person and their whānau situation are represented on a whiteboard diagram under a range of headings. This tool encompasses Māori understandings about identity, wairua, and intergenerational family processes alongside contemporary psychiatric considerations such as biological, psychological, and social factors that may be contributing to the young person and their family's predicament.

References

American Psychiatric Association. (2013) *Diagnostic and statistical manual of mental disorders*, DSM-5 (5th edn). American Psychiatric Association, Arlington.

Barnes, A. (2013) 'What can Pākehā learn from engaging in kaupapa Māori educational research?' Working Paper 1. NZ Council for Educational Research, Wellington.

Cherrington, L. (2002) 'The use of Māori mythology in clinical settings: Training issues and needs'. Proceedings of the National Māori Graduates of Psychology Symposium, Waikato.

Durie, M. (1998) *Whaiora: Māori health development* (2nd edn). Oxford University Press, Melbourne.

———. (2003) *Ngā Kāhui Pou: Launching Māori Futures*. Huia, Wellington.

———. (2009) 'Maori knowledge and medical science: The interface between psychiatry and traditional healing in New Zealand'. Chapter 19 in Incayawar, M., Wintrob, R. & Bouchard, L. (eds), *Psychiatrists and traditional healers: Unwitting partners in global mental health*, pp. 237–49. John Wiley & Sons, Chichester.

Durie, M., Milroy, H. & Hunter, E. (2009) 'Mental health and the indigenous peoples of Australia and New Zealand'. Chapter 2 in Kirmayer, L. & Valaskakis, G. (eds), *Healing traditions: The mental health of aboriginal peoples in Canada*, pp. 36–55. University of British Columbia Press, Vancouver.

McCreanor, T. (2012) 'Challenging and countering anti-Māori discourse: Practices for decolonisation'. Chapter 15 in Nairn, R., Pehi, P., Black, R. & Waitoki, W. (eds), *Ka Tū, Ka Oho: Visions of a bicultural partnership in psychology*, pp. 289–310. NZ Psychological Society, Wellington.

Mila, K. (2014) 'Mana Moana'. Unpublished manuscript.

Nairn, M. (2002) 'Decolonisation for Pākehā'. In Margaret, J. (ed.), *Pākehā Treaty work: Unpublished material*, pp. 203–06. Manukau Institute of Technology Treaty Unit, Auckland.

Ngata, H.M. (1993) *English–Maori dictionary*. Learning Media, Wellington.

Ruha, P. (2007) 'Te pounamu: An introduction'. Unpublished manuscript.

Sadock, B.J. & Sadock, V.A. (2005) *Kaplan and Sadock's comprehensive textbook of psychiatry* (8th edn). Lippincott Williams & Wilkins, New York.

Satir, V. & Baldwin, M. (1983) *Satir step by step: A guide to creating change in families*. Science and Behaviour Books, Palo Alto.

Sims, A. (1995) *Symptoms in the mind: An introduction to descriptive psychopathology* (2nd edn). Saunders, London.

Smith, L.T. (2012) *Decolonizing methodologies: Research and indigenous peoples* (2nd edn). Otago University Press, Dunedin.

Tamasese, T.K. (2012) 'Interface of gender and culture'. Chapter 1 in Nairn, R., Pehi, P., Black, R. & Waitoki, W. (eds), *Ka Tū, Ka Oho: Visions of a bicultural partnership in psychology*, pp. 31–38. NZ Psychological Society, Wellington.

Waldegrave, C., Tamasese, K., Tuhaka, F. & Campbell, W. (2003) *Just Therapy- a journey: A collection of papers from the Just Therapy Team, New Zealand*. Dulwich Centre Publications, Adelaide.

Watters, E. (2010) *Crazy like us: The globalization of the American psyche*. Free Press, New York.

GLOSSARY

āhua—appearance
Aotearoa[1]—Māori name for New Zealand
aroha—love
awa—river/rivers
fa'asamoa (Samoan)—Samoan worldview
hākari—feast, banquet
hapū—subtribe
hīkoi—a walk or journey
Hineahuone—the earth maiden
hinengaro—mind/psychological
Hinenuitepō—the maiden of darkness, death and the underworld
Hinetītama—the dawn maiden
hōhā—annoyed
hongi—to press noses in greeting
hua—fruit, product
Io—supreme being, God
iwi—tribe
kai—food
kaiako—teacher
kaimahi—clinician or worker
kāinga—home, village
kaitiaki—guardian, guardians
kapahaka—Māori cultural group
karakia—prayer/prayers or ritual chant
karanga—to call; formal or ceremonial call
kaumātua—elder/elders
kaupapa Māori—Māori approach

kāwanatanga—governance, government
kawemate—bereavement ceremony sometime after the burial of the deceased person
kēhua—ghost, spirit that remains nearby after death
kei te pai—it's okay/I'm okay
kete—basket
kina—sea urchin
koro—elderly man/grandfather
koroua—elderly man/grandfather
kōrero—conversation, talk, explanation
korowai—cloak, traditionally a fine feather cloak
kōtiro—girl
kuia—female elder, grandmother
kupu—word
mahi—work
mahi wairua—spiritual healing work
maki tūpāpaku (Cook Islands Māori)—form of spirit possession
mākutu—an act intended to cause physical or psychological harm via use of spiritual powers
mana—spiritual authority
manaakitanga—to support, give hospitality, show respect and generosity to others
manuhiri—visitors
Māori/māori—indigenous person of Aotearoa (New Zealand)/normal or usual
marae—Māori meeting house. Also the open area in front of the meeting house where formal greetings and discussions take place
matai (Samoan)—titled head or chief of a Samoan family
matakite—seer/foresight
mate Māori—Māori sickness or illness
matekite—seer of sickness or death
Māui—Māori demigod, also known as Māui-pōtiki and Māui-tikitiki-a-Taranga
mauri—life force
mihi—greeting
mihi whakatau—speeches of welcome, round of introductions
moana—sea/ocean
moko—short for mokopuna (grandchild)
moko—Māori facial tattoo
moko kauae—Māori chin tattoo worn traditionally by elder women
mokopuna—grandchild, grandchildren
muru—ritual compensation, restorative justice
ngaro—lost
ngāwari—kind, flexible, affable, easy-going
noa—free from tapu
Pākehā—New Zealander of European descent

pālagi (Samoan)—person of European descent
papa kāinga—home base, village, birth place
Papatūānuku—Earth Mother
pepe—baby
pepeha—saying, introduction
pito—umbilical cord
poi—light ball on a string twirled rhythmically in song, kapahaka art form
pounamu—New Zealand greenstone or jade, greenstone pendant or precious object
pōwhiri—ceremonial welcome
rākau—stick, ceremonial staff
rangatahi—adolescent
rangatiratanga—unqualified authority, sovereignty
Ranginui—God of the sky and husband of Papatūānuku
rāpaki—a traditional garment worn from the waist to the knees
raruraru—trouble, conflict
rongoā—herbal medicinal preparations
taiaha—spear shaped weapon
take—cause
tamariki—children
tā moko—Māori tattooing on the face or body using traditional protocols
Tānenuiārangi—Māori demigod who ascended the heavens to collect the three baskets of knowledge, son of Ranginui and Papatūānuku
tangata whaiora—clients, or mental health service users; literally: people seeking health
tangata whenua—indigenous people of the land
tangi—bereavement ritual, short for tangihanga
taonga—something precious which may be tangible or intangible
ta'unga (Cook Islands Māori)—traditional healer
tapu—to be sacred, restricted or forbidden
Taranga—mother of Māui
tarutaru—cannabis, weeds
tātaihono—spiritual binding together that confers unity and strength to a partnership
taumaha—heaviness
te ao Māori—the Māori world, or worldviews
te ao wairua—the spiritual realm
Te Kaihanga—the creator, God
Tēnā koutou katoa—hello, a greeting addressed to three or more people
te reo Māori—the Māori language
Te Whare Mārie—literally, the house of peace: Māori mental health service based in Porirua
te taha hinengaro—the psychological side or part
te taha tinana—the physical side

te taha wairua—the spiritual side
te taha whānau—the family or relational side
tiakitanga—guardianship
tikanga—correct procedure or convention, usually referring to Māori customs
tikitiki—topknot of hair
tinana—body, physical
tīpuna, tūpuna—ancestors
tohunga—Māori traditional healer or expert
tohunga wānanga—tohunga centre/centres of learning
tūpāpaku—body of deceased person
tūrangawaewae—literally 'place to stand', refers to a person's ancestral lands
tūrehu—spiritual creatures that are part human and part animal
urupā—cemetery, burial ground
utu—reciprocity, cost, may also be revenge
waewae tapu—newcomer, person who has not been to a particular marae before
wahine—woman
waiata—song, songs
waiora—health, well-being
wairua—spiritual, spirituality
wairuatanga—spirituality
wānanga—Māori tertiary education institution, seminar
whaikōrero—formal speech, oratory
whaiora—seeker of wellbeing, client, patient
whaiwhaiā—being pursued spiritually
whakaiti—to make oneself small, be humble
whakamana—to give authority or prestige to, to enhance the mana of another/others
whakanoa—make free from tapu
whakapapa—genealogy
whakatauākī—proverb
whakawetewete—ritual to resolve conflict, hurt or transgressions between people
whānau—family
whare—house
whatumanawa—deep-seated emotions
whenua—land; also afterbirth or placenta

Note

1. The definitions in this glossary come from Wiremu and a variety of other sources but we are particularly indebted to the online Māori Dictionary accessed at https://maoridictionary.co.nz for guidance on many of the definitions.

NGĀ MIHI (ACKNOWLEDGEMENTS)

E tuku mihi nei ki Te Kaihanga mō ōna manaakitanga.[1]

Me ngā mihi hoki ki ngā rangatahi me ō rātou whānau mō tā rātou tautoko ki tēnei kaupapa me ngā whakaaetanga kia oti atu i a mātou tēnei pukapuka. Me te mīharo ki ngā kōrero, ngā whakaaro, ngā āwangawanga me ngā mamae, tangi me ngā huarahi i kitea e rātou. Kei te mihi, kei te mihi, kei te mihi. E whai whakaaro ana ki ngā mātua tīpuna, nā rātou i toro te nukuroa kia taea e tātou te whai ake i ngā mātauranga kia kitea he huarahi mō tātou te tangata. Ki a rātou kia mene ki te kohinga wairua.

Ka haere tonu ngā mihi ki ngā mana whenua a Toa Rangatira. Tēnā koutou, tēnā koutou, tēnā koutou.

Ko ngā kaumātua me ngā pou o Te Whare Mārie, tēnā koutou.

Ko taku tuahine te kirituna, mai te whānau a Hinekōrako, kei te mihi.

Ko taku rangatira, mai Ngā Kurī-a-Whārei ki Tihirau, kei te mihi.

Ki ngā toa e mahi ana i roto i te kaupapa kei Te Whare tonu koutou, kua wehe atu rānei ki mahi kē, tēnei te mihi nui, tēnā koutou, tēnā koutou, tēnā koutou katoa.

Ki ngā iwi taketake, ngā whanaunga mai ngā moutere o Te Moana-nui-a-Kiwa, tēnā koutou.

Meitaki maata ki te au Kopu Tangata, te au Mapu, te Ui Tupuna, i te Ipukarea o te Cook Islands.[2]

Fa'afetai tele i le lotomau ma lo outou finagalo tatala.[3]

We especially acknowledge the courage and generosity of the young people and family members who gave consent and approval for their stories to be shared. Without them this book could not have been written. We also acknowledge our guides and mentors: those who have passed on and those who are still with us, who shared their wisdom and inspired our exploration of these less described territories of experience. They include Te Awhimate Trainor NiaNia, Huatahi NiaNia, Hohepa Kereopa, Rua Kēnana, Pikau Te Rangi Arthur, Ani Tangiwai Sweet, Bill (Paul) Cox, Dr Thakshan Fernando, Dr Howard Cooper, Taimalieutu Kiwi Tamasese, Charles Waldegrave, and Michael White. We also acknowledge the significant contribution of His Highness Tui Atua Tupua Tamasese Efi to the interface between Western science and indigenous knowledge.

Thank you to Lesley NiaNia, Ruth Diggins, and Ann Epston for their unswerving support and belief in this project and Pastor Norm McLeod for his guidance.

We thank all our colleagues at Te Whare Mārie and Health Pasifika, past and present, who have advocated passionately for wairua to be addressed in our mental health services and contributed directly or indirectly to the mahi described in this book. Although many colleagues influenced our thinking, we acknowledge the leadership of mana whenua with Te Wera Kotua, Tai Elkington, and Jayne Isaacs; the tautoko of Kui Mere Hammond; the foundations laid by Peta Ruha; the outspoken advocacy of Hinengakau Taurerewa and Egan Bidois; and the support of Faamausili Chapman, Folole Esera, and Mercy Drummond.

We are grateful to Gay Puketapu-Andrews, Wakaiti Saba, Dr Evangelene Daniela, Tafaoimalo Loudeen Parsons, and Professor Lady Arohia Durie for their perceptive comments on cultural matters in particular chapters. We thank Dr Karlo Mila for detailed suggestions which enhanced several chapters and the final title. Dr Tim McCreanor and Robert Consedine provided valued responses on historical and social science matters in the text. We thank Cathy Diggins, James Bush, Richard Sawrey, Craig Whisker, Rachel Hayward, Liz O'Connor, Professor Stephen Robertson, Dr Robyn Blake, Brian Archer, Virginia Tatton, John Tovey, Cheryl White, David Denborough, and other colleagues, friends, and whānau members whose astute comments have sharpened our thinking and improved the book.

This book won first prize in the Ashton Wylie Charitable Trust (AWCT) Unpublished Manuscript Award in 2014. We are very appreciative of this financial support and the encouragement from AWCT members, and judges Bob Ross and Mary Egan. We also acknowledge Capital Coast District Health Board for supporting the sabbatical period that enabled the completion of the manuscript.

We are very grateful to Mitch Allen and Art Bochner at Left Coast Press who believed in this project and guided us over several years. We thank our New Zealand editor, Gillian Tewsley, for her careful attention to improving the manuscript and Hannah Shakespeare and the team at Routledge for their support and assistance with the publication of this book.

We owe a debt of gratitude to our psychiatrist advisors: Drs Bridget Taumoepeau, Joanna MacDonald, Alec MacDonald, and Professor Pete Ellis, who reviewed all the chapters, and Drs Liam O'Connor, Leeanne Fisher, Susan Perry, Richard Holt, Kristin Sparks, Philippa Loan, and Professor Sarah Romans for comments on particular chapters. While we thank each of them for their contribution, any errors are the responsibility of the authors.

Finally we acknowledge our moko tuarua (great-grandchildren), mokopuna (grandchildren), tamariki (children), and the many other tamariki that we would call our own. They are an expression of our whakapapa and they are our future. They inspire us to reflect on how we can best whakamana young people everywhere.

We finish with this whakatauākī:

> Ehara taku toa i te toa takitahi, engari he toa takitini.
> To acknowledge this mahi is to acknowledge all the people who stand with us.

Notes

1. In this passage in te reo Māori we acknowledge our creator who sustains us, the young people, and their families who generously gave their stories and all those who came before us. We acknowledge the people of Ngāti Toa Rangatira who are the traditional owners of the land where Te Whare Mārie stands, the kaumātua and kaimahi of Te Whare Mārie, and all our friends and colleagues from the Pacific who have contributed to this book.
2. In this passage in the Cook Islands language we offer sincere thanks to the Cook Islands families, the young people, the ancestors, and the land from which they came, the Cook Islands.
3. This passage in the Samoan language offers a heartfelt acknowledgement of the contribution of the Samoan families and colleagues who supported the development of this book.

INDEX